Lose Weight, Have More Energy & Be Happier in 10 Days

Take charge of your health with the Master Cleanse

By Peter Glickman

Lose Weight, Have More Energy & Be Happier in 10 Days
© 2004, 2005, 2010, 2011, 2015 by Peter Glickman, Inc.

First Edition, August 2004
Second Edition, March 2005
Third Edition, January 2011
Fourth Edition, April 2015

Published by Peter Glickman, Inc., 2251 Willowbrook Drive,
Clearwater, Florida 33764.

Editing, design and layout by Maggy Graham

Illustrations by Ann Khotina

Indexing by Rossinna Ippolito, inDocs inDexing Services

Publisher's Cataloging-in-Publication Data

Glickman, Peter
        Lose weight, have more energy & be happier in 10 days
    / Peter Glickman.—4th ed.—Clearwater, FL: Peter Glickman,
2015.
        192 p. 21.6 cm.
        ISBN 978-0-9755722-5-2
        1. Diet Therapy Popular Works. 2. Juice Diet. I. Title.
    RM237.G55 2004   615.854'22

Printed in the United States of America.

THE INFORMATION GIVEN IN THIS BOOK IS SOLELY FOR
EDUCATIONAL PURPOSES. IT IS NOT INTENDED AS MEDICAL
ADVICE. ANYONE WHO FOLLOWS IT DOES SO VOLUNTARILY.

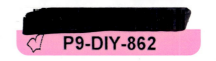

Testimonials

"In August, I was diagnosed with a brain tumor. Most days are filled with headaches, dizziness, nausea, and some visual/balance problems. I've never had regular bowel movements and have always had bloating, gas, and several problems because of that. Since starting the cleanse, all those symptoms have disappeared and I've lost twelve pounds. I'm completely thrilled!! I go back to the neurologist Monday and can't wait to tell him all this.

"I plan to eat much healthier (after breaking the fast appropriately). I have more energy and clarity and feel more like myself.

"I just wanted to give my 'testimony.' This has been a godsend."

—Angi Hardin

*****

"Peter, thanks again for the inspiration and information. I've lost about twelve to fourteen pounds. My waist is down two and one-half to three inches. I have to get another belt because the ones I have are all on the last notch. I've walked forty-six miles since starting, ridden my bike fourteen miles, and have worked each day (some better than others). I have a great feeling of peace, even though I hit some pretty stressful events head on. I am also giving serious thought to other work/life things. I guess the clarity and focus come from not eating. It is also a time to look at priorities."—Tony Bruno

*****

"I am a diabetic. I weighed 150 pounds six years ago before surgery on my right knee. Then an infection developed and I had intravenous antibiotics for several months. When I left the hospital, I weighed 230 pounds and had diabetes. None of the doctors or specialists could restore circulation in that leg. They referred me to a doctor for an amputation, but I refused to give up the leg. I sought treatment with a chiropractor who did Contact Reflex Analysis and restored circulation that same day. He put me on a protein-only diet. I put away the crutches and went back to work.

"Now, years later, I was dreading going to work as I hurt so badly. It was a struggle to keep ahead of the assembly line. I am 64 years old and was 188 pounds. My co-workers are half my age. We work as a team, but I was not doing my part. My shoulders just couldn't lift a hammer. My elbows hurt. My wrists wouldn't bend and my fingers were swollen. By the end of the workday, my feet were burning like they were on fire and had become so swollen it was difficult to get them out of my work boots. My right knee had to be lubricated with olive oil twice during the work day or else my skin stuck to my knee cap and I fell down. This is because I had no lubricated membrane in my knee joint.

"I had a physical at work and they said my PSA [a chemical in blood that shows the risk for prostate cancer in men] had jumped from .6 to 6.4 and that I needed to check it out further. I went to my family doctor to repeat the blood test and set an appointment. The doctor's office called me two days after the second test and said my appointment was changed to a specialist as the PSA came back at 14.6!

"After a biopsy showed all was OK, I asked the doctor if I could do a colon cleanse and a fast before the next appointment. He said 'That's sounds like something my mother would do, but it would be fine.'

"I had bought *Prostate Health in 90 Days* by Larry Clapp and it prescribed Stanley Burroughs' cleanse, except that Larry used twice as much lemonade daily (16 glasses) and also bentonite & psyllium to help flush the system. It was an eight-day detox. My first day on the cleanse there was no shoulder pain, my elbows no longer hurt, I could work without the wrist supports and the finger swelling went away! Something was going on. When I got home from work and got out of the truck my legs and feet worked and I no longer had to shuffle into the house like a ninety-year-old man.

"During these eight days I was looking for more information and I found your website. I discovered that it was Stanley Burroughs' plan and that there was more information. You were there to educate me and even had a support group.

"I had decided to do forty days as that was the maximum time recommended. You even advised me to cut my cleanse short as it was my first, but I felt good—really good—so I continued. At work, I started accepting overtime and never got tired, light-headed, hyper, or hungry. I craved nothing, but wanted everything!

"The first week I lost no weight, but many inches everywhere. I had been wearing size 36 jeans, but my stomach hung over a little. My physical said I had a 42-inch waist. After my second week, my stomach disappeared, but the skin sagged down to my groin. During the third week, my foot pain went away as well as the swelling that made it hard to remove my work boots. I was no longer rubbing castor oil on my feet day and night.

"About the same time, my big toe, that won't bend because of gout, was now bending and is without pain. It's still swollen, as the bones seem to have calcium deposits, but it works fine. In the fourth week, my right knee began working fine with no need for external lubrication. Oh, I still favor it, but it's fine even going up or down steps.

"In my fifth week, I can't help but notice that my toenails need cutting. Previously, I cut my toenails twice a year, but they never seemed to grow. Now, they are growing as fast as my finger nails.

"While on the cleanse, I checked my blood sugar. During the second week of the cleanse, it started to elevate to 140, so I cut back two ounces of maple syrup and my blood sugar dropped to 70. [He was making up six drinks at a time.] That was too low, so I increased it by one ounce to five ounces and it leveled off at 100. In Week 4 it increased again to 140, so I cut back to four ounces and kept it there till I finished the forty days.

"Today is my second day on solid food and it is my intent to minimize animal products, but this is another lifestyle change and will take some getting used to. My tongue is still white. I now weigh 160 lbs and do not hang over my 32-inch jeans. There are wrinkles leading out in every direction from my belly button and I am cold all the time. One-third of my forty days were good days. The rest were sad, depressed or neutral, but each day was different and I had the strength to face them.

"All in all, it has been an enjoyable fast. I am so thankful for your encouragement and the help of your book. I thought I was alone."

—Dick Maslowski

Table of Contents

A Huge Debt x

Confession xi

Foreword xiii

Introduction xv

Part I: Perspective..1

    Current Health Care Statistics...2

    Ideas in Conflict 4

    Challenging Established Authority...4

    Support for Alternative Medicine 6

    America's Health Crisis 7

Part II: Anti-Aging 2

    Scientific Studies 9

    A More Practical Approach 11

    The Chicken Heart that Lived Forever 12

    My Experience with the Master Cleanse 13

    What About Protein, Vitamins and Minerals?....................14

    The Future...15

Part III: How to Do the Master Cleanse.........................16

    Shopping List..16

    Quick Start 17

    More Details..19

    For Those with Diabetes or High Blood Pressure 25

    Detox Symptoms—the Good, the Bad and the Ugly 26

    "How About Only Five Days? Can We Make a Deal?"........30

    The Agitator and the Rinse Cycle.......................................31

    The Master Cleanse is Not for Everyone 32

    If Detox Symptoms Become Unpleasant 34

Table of Contents

Headaches 35

When It Is Not All Coming Out as Planned 35

The Twelve Most Common Pitfalls 36

What to Expect Day by Day 40

The Detox Diet Scale 42

Part IV: Your Master Cleanse Journal 44

Part V: The Master Cleanse Discussion Bulletin Board 45

Acid/Alkaline Balance/pH? 45

After the Cleanse 46

Agave Nectar vs. Maple Syrup 48

Anti-depressants 49

Bentonite, Psyllium, Herbs, Colon Cleansers
During the Cleanse 49

Beyond 10 Days 51

Boredom 52

Bowel Movements 54

Bowel Movements Not Happening 60

Breaking the Fast—Very Important 63

Bronchitis, Asthma 65

Brushing Your Teeth During the Cleanse 66

Candida 66

Cayenne Pepper 67

Cheating—Am I Alone? 68

Chemotherapy, Cancer and the Cleanse 70

Chewing Gum 71

Cleansing, Other Types 71

Cold, Feeling 72

Colonics 73

Cramping 74

Cravings 74

Daily Experiences 75

Day 1 81

Day 3—Feeling Good 83

Day 5 85

Day 10! 86
Diabetics, Special Instructions 88
Diarrhea...88
Emotional Detox?...89
Emotional Eating...90
Exercise, Running, and Weights 90
Friends and Family 90
Hair Loss 91
Headaches on the Cleanse...91
Health—Attitudes About...92
Hemorrhoids 93
High Blood Pressure...93
Honey vs. Maple Syrup 93
Hunger vs. Cravings...94
Hypoglycemia/Low Blood Sugar 95
Infertility and the Cleanse 95
Interrupting the Cleanse 96
Intestinal/Abdominal Cramps 96
January Cleanse...96
Laxative Tea 101
Lemonade, Amount to Drink 102
Lemonade, Premixing 103
Lemons, Buying in Quantity 104
Lemons, Juicing..104
Length of Cleanses and Time Between Them.................106
Madal Bal Syrup/Neera Cleanse......................................107
Maple Syrup, Loving It a Little Too Much 108
Maple Syrup Substitute..109
Maple Syrup, Unable to Handle the Taste of 110
Master Cleanse Beginner 111
Master Cleanse Book, Pass It Along.................................113
Medication 115
Minerals...118
Mucoid Plaque 118

Table of Contents

Nothing Happening 120

Osteoporosis 127

Other Cleanses—Liver/Kidney/Parasite Cleanse 128

Pain 128

Parasites 125

Passing Gas—Warning 131

Personal Health, Observations On 131

Pregnant, Trying to Get 132

Protein—a Raw Vegetarian Diet and Weight Lifting 134

Quitting on Detox Days 135

Running or Exercising During the Diet 136

Salt Water Flush 137

Sea Salt with Iodine 142

Skin 142

Sleeping Patterns 142

Smoking, Quitting During the Cleanse 143

Spiritual Breakthrough 144

Starvation—Isn't This Starving Yourself? 145

Supplements 145

Surgery and the MC 145

Tea, Other Kinds 146

Time Between Cleanses—How Soon Can I Do It Again? 146

Tingling or Pain in the Teeth 147

Tongue Coating 147

Underweight 150

Vegetarian Diet 150

Water Fast Only 151

Weight Loss 152

Women's Issues 156

Word of Mouth 158

Afterword 160

References 161

Index 163

A Huge Debt

The original book on the Master Cleanse is *The Master Cleanser* by Stanley Burroughs. Without Burroughs' work and that book, mankind would be significantly poorer. His book describes the Master Cleanse along with his views on disease and healing, some natural remedies, and some recipes for healthy food. It can be purchased from the Web Store of my website, www. TheMasterCleanse.com.

Stanley Burroughs first published *The Master Cleanser* in 1976 and has sold hundreds of thousands of copies without advertising because of results. This new wave of attention will succeed provided it stays true to the original, time-tested Burroughs method. In coaching thousands of people, I have seen many variations, but the method that works best for most people is the original method. So, even if you have good results with a variation a time or two, please remember that the method with the greatest success for the most people is the original and pass along only that one. I owe a debt of gratitude to Stanley Burroughs and I hope when you are done you will too.

I am also in debt to all the wonderful people who participated on our bulletin board. Their encouragement, willingness to share, and insights have been and are wonderful, as you will see.

! NOTE: Throughout this book, an exclamation point to the left indicates the section is important.

Confession

I'm just an average Joe. I came upon the Master Cleanse because I was pig-headed enough to keep looking for a natural way to handle my failing health that would not cost me an arm and a leg and would not cause unwanted side effects. I just decided to keep looking until I found that way. Fortunately for me, I succeeded.

I am not a licensed health professional and cannot diagnose or prescribe. However, I knew what it had done for me in 2003 and I began to tell others on the Internet. There I saw the Master Cleanse help more than 100 people regain and maintain their vibrant good health in our first ever group Master Cleanse in January 2004. I also saw that people had the same questions over and over. So, I decided to write this book to answer those questions. Since then I have been fortunate enough to see literally thousands of people benefit from it. In just the month of January 2009, more than 1,200 people informed me they were doing the Master Cleanse!

From reading some of the great healers of the past, I believe people can extend their lives and avoid illness and disease if they eat mostly real, live food (raw fruits and vegetables, seeds and nuts), drink unpolluted and unfluoridated water, and clean their colons frequently.

I firmly believe that each person is responsible for his or her own health. If you want to be healthy, have energy and feel good, you must learn what is involved and apply it. You have to monitor what goes into your mouth, what exercise you do, what air you breathe, and most important of all, what thoughts you think. And you need to detoxify regularly.

The good news is that valuable knowledge is available if you take the time to look for it and are willing to determine if The Master Cleanse is true for you and your body. The reason you have to determine it for yourself is that each person's body is potentially different. For example, most people find penicillin valuable for killing bacteria. Some people are allergic and can die from it.

You are the only person who can make the determination of what is useful or not for you. Health professionals can give you valuable information and do other wonderful things, but ultimately, the buck stops with you. So you have to learn to use good judgment along with your experience, and that includes determining if the information in this book is useful to you.

Therefore, the information in this book is solely for educational purposes. It is not intended as medical advice or to diagnose, treat, cure or prescribe. If you decide to follow it, it must be because you have determined that it would be good for you to try it.

Each person should seek the counsel of their health professional, and then use his or her own judgment. This caution applies to the information in this book and that posted on the website—**www.TheMasterCleanse.com**. In fact, this caution applies to any information in life.

If you are in ill health, have any disease or are taking any medications and want to do the Master Cleanse, consult your licensed healthcare professional first. Most especially, do not discontinue any medications without guidance from a licensed healthcare professional.

I think the Master Cleanse is great. You have to decide for yourself. I am only telling my story and some of the many stories I have heard and read. If you have made the decision to do the Master Cleanse, congratulations for doing something really wonderful for yourself and your body!

Best wishes for your vibrant good health,

Peter Glickman

Foreword

Health care reform is a gargantuan issue facing not just the U.S. but also the entire world. I, too, believe that our system is broken and in need of change. However, I think Washington is barking up the wrong tree. They are busy arguing about coverage and access for the current "sick care" system when what the country truly needs is "health care" reform: reform that shifts the focus from a symptom-suppression model of sick care to one of prevention, wellness and the elimination of unnecessary drugs.

Ironically, Washington appears to mirror the problems that exist in Western Medicine. Sick care treats symptoms instead of dealing with the root causes of disease. Western medicine is not the medicine of the future because it does not address why we are unhealthy and how to change. If we do not change why we are unhealthy, we will continue to be unhealthy and we will remain economically distressed. To provide better health care, to become a healthier nation, we have to make serious changes. We will only flourish when we address the root causes of the problems.

For 2,200 years until 1805, medicine was practiced exclusively according to the ancient Greek physician Hippocrates (460-377 BC), the founding father of natural medicine. He taught that the first and foremost principal of medicine must be to respect nature's healing forces, which inhabit each living organism. Thus you are the only person who can cure yourself. Healers only assist. Hippocrates considered illness a natural phenomenon that forced people to discover the imbalances in their health. He strongly believed in good food and related the course of any disease to poor nutrition and bad eating habits. He taught, "Let food be your medicine and medicine be your food," advice that, to this day, has not lost its validity.

During the 1800s, a new school of medicine emerged: the allopathic school (using drugs to suppress the symptoms of a disease) or Western school, based on patentable drugs. The idea behind it was that doctors can cure, provided they have the correct technology and drugs. During this era, there were more homeopathic doctors (using natural substances to cure the disease) than allopathic ones, as they were preferred. However, by the 1920s, there was only one homeopathic school remaining. Motivated by profit and through legislative maneuvering, pharmaceutical giants ensured allopathic medical dominance, while ignoring the first rule of medicine: first do no harm. Thus, today we are offered drugs that treat depression with a side effect of suicide!

The reality is that medicine has failed to evolve while people are demanding change. No one seems to get well and cries from consumers fall upon deaf ears.

So, unfortunately, it is left up to you to navigate our unfortunate system of sick care. So for those seeking assistance, I relate a fact known for several thousand years: most illness comes from the colon. Few remember that at one time, colon therapists were an integral part of the general medical practice in America. Dr. John H Kellogg published: "Should the colon be sacrificed or may it be reformed?" in the *Journal of the American Medical Association*, Vol. 26 in 1917. After this publication, colon therapy grew in popularity in America until the invention of colonoscopy. Keeping your colon clean and healthy was replaced with simply looking at it.

As part of prevention, keeping your colon clean and healthy is of prime importance. That is one of the reasons the Master Cleanse is a great tool for those seeking prevention of illness and I respect Peter for doing a great job of not only explaining what to do, but also sharing with you others' experiences and support. Great health does not have to be expensive.

When I started my clinic, Utopia Wellness, I was tired of issuing bandaids in an effort to treat symptoms. I had to teach myself that real medicine is more than just technology and drugs. I became a physician because I wanted to help people find remedies for their problems. I wanted it to serve as a model for this necessary change in health care, where just about any disease is addressed naturally. We stress prevention, not intervention or sick care. Sick care is ineffective and expensive.

Perhaps someday, individuals who understand real health care for our nation may represent WE THE PEOPLE. In the mean time, you had better learn how to prevent illness, since there appears to be little profit for others to do so.

Carlos M. Garcia, M.D.
www.UtopiaAwaits.com

Introduction

November 1, 2010

In the fall of 2005, shortly after the second edition was published, I discovered that it was beneficial to take probiotics after the cleanse. and began to promote that on the Internet. (See number seven in the section "More Details" on page 24.) It has since been copied on the many thousands of websites offering advice on the Master Cleanse. However, that information never made it into this book. So I made a promise to myself that I would do a third edition.

The number of webpages discussing the Master Cleanse since the first edition is now almost half a million! This has led some people to accuse me of just copying whatever information I found on the Internet. I find this accusation funny considering there were less than a handful of websites devoted to the Master Cleanse when I wrote the first edition and put up the first Internet Bulletin Board (or forum, as they are called these days) at the end of 2003 and personally posted more than 600 answers to people's questions.

In the first and second edition I answered the 70 most frequently asked questions. Since then, the most frequently asked questions have changed a bit and answering those new questions was another reason I wanted to write this third edition.

I also wanted to publish at least a few of the many scientific studies that validate the Master Cleanse as I am frequently asked for that information by those who would like to spread the word.

My final reason for writing this third edition is the information on anti-aging, which I personally find fascinating and is directly related to the Master Cleanse and fasting. Fasting from time to time (intemittent fasting) and a permanent, restricted-calorie diet with optimum nutrition are the only two methods that have ever been scientifically proven to extend life and reduce the diseases of aging! (See the section "Anti-Aging".)

Being overweight has become far too common in America. According to a *Business Week* article, ("Those Heavy Americans," Gene Koretz,

Business Week, Nov. 10, 2003) two-thirds of Americans are overweight. The market for weight loss products (low carbohydrate foods, diet programs, reducing supplements, etc.) was projected to surpass $150 billion by 2007.[1]

Still worse, obesity or being overweight was the third leading cause of preventable death in the United States from 2003–2006.[2] Those people it does not kill, it punishes, especially dating singles who want to be attractive to the opposite sex.

A look at our current culture might provide an explanation. *Super Size Me* is a very entertaining, feature-length color documentary film that shows what happens when the central character actually goes on a 30-day McDonald's-only diet. For 30 days, he eats breakfast, lunch and dinner at McDonald's. Nothing passes his lips that cannot be purchased at McDonald's. And whenever they ask him if he wants it super-sized, he must answer yes and eat it all.

At the beginning of the movie, we see him getting the results of various examinations by health care professionals. His results are all normal and he is given a clean bill of health. After three weeks, one doctor is shocked at how much worse his liver is and encourages him to go off the diet. Our "dieter" refuses. So, the doctor hands him a number for the hospital emergency room and insists he call if he experiences any symptoms of a heart attack! The doctor is shown in the film saying something along the lines of, "I would never have imagined that your diet could reduce your health this fast."

Not only does he gain more weight than expected, but we watch the deterioration in his complexion and mental attitude as well as learn about it from the results of his later blood tests. There are segments where he talks about his worsened mental attitude. His girlfriend, a vegan chef, also talks about his diminished sexual capability. (So, do not show the entire movie to your six year old without seeing it first. His girlfriend's description is not graphic, but you may have to answer questions you would rather not, if you show that part to your six year old.)

---

1   "Weight Loss Market: Products, Services, Foods and Beverages," Business Communications Co., Inc., Aug. 7, 2003

2   "The Preventable Causes of Death in the United States: Comparative Risk Assessment of Dietary, Lifestyle, and Metabolic Risk Factors," Public Library of Science–Medicine, 2009

Another scene shows how children with learning and attitude problems change for the better when they are not fed processed food in their school cafeteria.

Toward the end of the movie, McDonald's French fries, a hamburger and a sandwich are put in separate glass domes along with a fresh-ground hamburger and hand-cut French fries from a local restaurant. The fresh-ground hamburger and hand-cut French fries decomposed as you would expect because they are not refrigerated. However, even without refrigeration, the McDonald's fries have no visible decomposition even after six weeks!

If they do not decompose like "nutritional" food, what does your body do with them? Your body uses the food you eat to nourish your body & blood, and build new cells. When you eat something that contains artificial preservatives, colors or flavors, your body has to neutralize it before it is eliminated. This is one of the jobs of the liver. When the liver receives too much to process at the time, it stores those toxins in fat cells in the liver to process later. When the liver runs out of room to store these, it releases them into the body and the body creates fat cells and stores the toxins in the body's fat cells until the toxins can be processed.

What keeps your liver strong and healthy? Blood from the colon is fed directly to the liver to nourish it. However, the body accumulates uneliminated toxins especially in the large intestine (colon), where blood has to filter through these toxins and poisons to get to the liver. At this point, the whole body is being fed "dirty blood." This is like trying to wash your hands in paint to get them clean. This is also what medicine refers to as "autointoxication": not "intoxication" as in happily relaxed, but as in self-poisoned.[3]

Symptoms of autointoxication include headaches, nausea, mental depression, irritability, stress, tension, tiredness, sluggishness, mental fogginess, indecision, insomnia, and susceptibility to other illnesses.

It is the toxins that Americans are eating and drinking that ares causing the epidemic of overweight. Our bodies cannot handle the volume of toxins we consume on a daily basis.

---

3 *Tissue Cleansing Through Bowel Management,* Bernard Jensen, DC, ND, Ph.D., 1980

Think processed food does not have toxins? In the article "Why McDonald's Fries Taste So Good,"[4] the author, Eric Schlosser, says "About 90 percent of the money that Americans now spend on food goes to buy processed food." He goes on to say that the flavor is replaced with chemicals to add flavor. For example, there are approximately 350 different chemicals in high-quality artificial strawberry flavor.

Further in his article, he says, "One of the most widely used color additives ..., cochineal [pronounced koash-a-neil] extract ... is made from the [dried] bodies of [a small] female ... insect harvested mainly in Peru and the Canary Islands. The bug feeds on red cactus berries, and color from the berries accumulates in the females and their unhatched [young]. The insects are collected, dried, and ground into a pigment. It takes about 70,000 of them to produce a pound of carmine, which is used to make processed foods look pink, red, or purple. Dannon strawberry yogurt gets its color from carmine, and so do many frozen fruit bars, candies, and fruit fillings, and Ocean Spray pink-grapefruit juice drink."[5]

The artificial sweetener Aspartame, also sold as NutraSweet, Equal, Equal Measure, and Spoonful, is another good example. The Food and Drug Administration has a system that permits people to report bad health reactions to food and drugs. According to David Rietz's website (www.dorway.com), in February of 1994, Aspartame accounted for more than 75 percent of all bad reactions reported!

A *Plane and Pilot* magazine article from January 1990 on food additives explained that diet soft drinks are sweetened artificially by Aspartame (NutraSweet and Equal). Aspartame contains ten percent methanol, a poison, that is released at temperatures above 86° or if left on the shelf for a long time.

The article goes on to say that methanol destroys the brain a little at a time. Immediate effects can either be severe (epileptic seizures, blindness, or chest palpitations) or less noticeable (blurred vision, bright flashes, tunnel vision, ringing or buzzing in ears, migraine headaches, dizziness, loss of equilibrium, or lip and mouth reactions). It reports on an Air Force pilot who directly traced the patterns of tremors and seizures he suffered for two years to his consuming

---

4 "Why McDonald's Fries Taste So Good," Eric Schlosser, *The Atlantic Monthly,* Jan. 2001

5 "Why McDonald's Fries Taste So Good," Eric Schlosser, accessed at www.rense.com/general7/whyy.htm.

NutraSweet in beverages. His medical problems ceased when he quit drinking NutraSweet.

By the way, on 27 June 1996, without public notice, the FDA removed all restrictions from Aspartame, allowing it to be used in everything, including all heated and baked goods.[6]

Even when you go on a diet and eat less, forcing the body to burn fat, as soon as you go off the diet, the fat returns. The body must create more fat cells to protect itself from the toxins. The only effective way to eliminate the fat is to eliminate the toxins. This is why the Master Cleanse is so effective for not only losing weight, but also increasing energy and making people happier. In the informal survey of 141 people who have done or are on the Master Cleanse, about 80 percent of them report having more energy and more than 90 percent report being happier! This should be no surprise since toxins give you headaches, make you fell tired and irritable, and cause aches and pains. And the Master Cleanse, according to its developer, Stanley Burroughs, not only cleanses the colon, but also the liver, kidneys and other organs and glands.

A raw vegetable, fruit, seed and nut diet will also detoxify you, although more slowly. But in my experience, very, very few people can simply switch to eating 100 percent raw because their cravings overwhelm them and cause them to go off the raw food. However, a great many people can do the Master Cleanse and, having eliminated some cravings, eat a greater percentage of raw food than before. This is supported by the above survey, which showed that people on average rated their diet after the Master Cleanse as being somewhat healthier than before the Master Cleanse.

How did I learn about the Master Cleanse and the raw food diet? Well, in the fall of 1998, I was a successful executive of a small local software company. I was coming home at 6:30 pm and dropping into bed, so tired I did not even eat dinner. I would not get up until it was 8 a.m. and time to go to work again. No one at work, except my wife, knew I was not doing well. At home, however, my excessive tiredness and short temper were inescapable. Worse, food had become my enemy. No matter what I ate, I felt sick afterward.

About a year and a half before, I had been tested and discovered I had enough mercury in my body to interfere with normal system function. Apparently, it was finally getting to me. I sought a local

---

6 webhome.idirect.com / ~wolfnowl / aspartame.htm

doctor to do a mercury detoxification program on me and before he put me on that program, he gave me a thorough checkup.

The blood test came back with alarming numbers. My fasting blood sugar was in the range of diabetics (157), the fats that circulate in the bloodstream and are stored in the fat tissue (triglycerides) were really, really high (1160) and my cholesterol was in the same scary place (482). The doctor scared me badly enough that I radically changed my diet. I eliminated any sweet food including sweet fruits, sweet vegetables, etc. and added the vitamins and minerals that Adele Davis recommended for diabetics in her book, *Let's Get Well*. This was in addition to the mercury detoxification program, which included super greens (a combination of spirulina, blue green algae, alfalfa, wheatgrass and other greens).

Fortunately, in the next four months, my tests all returned to normal levels and I could go back to eating the standard American diet of too many fats, too much sugar, very few raw vegetables or fruits, and lots of processed food. Three years later in May 2002, I had another checkup and this time, although my fasting blood sugar was fine (108), my blood fats were the second highest the doctor had ever seen (1921) and my cholesterol was so scary (525) that he had his office call me in immediately to be put on a prescription. I listened to him, filled it immediately and tried it for three days. It gave me a headache and bad dreams. I figured I had licked the blood sugar problem with nutrition, why could I not lick the cholesterol problem the same way?

By May 2002, my wife had been eating a 100 percent raw fruit, vegetable, nuts and seeds diet for more than two months. She was looking healthy and radiant, had lost weight, had plenty of energy and felt great. I tried to ignore how healthy she was for several months, but after the prescription fiasco, I decided I would go on the same diet and see what happened. I was not feeling as bad as I had before the mercury detoxification; I still did not realize my road rage was connected to my health; and I still did not have the energy I used to have. But was that not normal?

When I started the raw vegetarian diet in May 2002, I weighed over 230 pounds. I wore pants with a size 40 waist, which were tight. Over the next six months, I lost more than thirty pounds and was now fitting into size 37 pants. But more importantly I felt great and had lots of energy. Road rage became a thing of the past. People who saw me asked what I was doing to look so much better.

In December 2002, I began wondering if I should do some kind of cleanse. I had done a liver/gall bladder cleanse some years before and wondered if perhaps another type of cleanse or a whole series of different cleanses was something I needed at this point. So when I discovered the Master Cleanse by Stanley Burroughs at the end of December, I decided to do it starting in January 2003.

The Master Cleanse changed my life. I did it for 20 days and lost 23 pounds. Much, much more important, I felt fabulous and was now able to work 10 – 14 hour days with no strain at all and I was happier than I had been in years and years!

My wife also did the Master Cleanse. So did my twenty-seven year old son and his girl friend, as well as a friend I had not seen in three years. When he heard I had lost over fifty pounds and felt great, he said he wanted to do it and did not care what it was. He discovered that on the Master Cleanse, he could still walk his six miles a day and he had enough energy to also ride his bike another four miles most days as well.

I already had a website for raw food and decided to add information on the Master Cleanse and a bulletin board so people who had questions could have a place to get answers from those who had done the Master Cleanse. From there, it was only a small step to see if we could get 100 people to do the Master Cleanse in January 2004 to start the year. Amazingly, with only one story in a local monthly health magazine and word of mouth, we ended up with more than 110 people doing it! That has increased to over 1200 in January of 2009!

Did I keep the weight off? That's a question I am frequently asked. Well, I finished my first Master Cleanse on 24 January

2003 weighing 175 pounds. For the next five years, doing three or four Master Cleanses a year, I stayed between 175 and 185. In October 2007, I began a program of research into the nature and laws of life that requires I eat every day and so I have not done a Master Cleanse since then. I look forward to finishing my research and again doing regular Master Cleanses. I am currently 200 pounds, but still in vibrant good health and it shows.

I wish you the best,
Peter Glickman

Part I:

First Things First

Perspective

The daughter of a friend of mine left for college this year. But first, my friend had a father-daughter talk with her. He did not like Bob, the boy she was dating at school. Bob did not have a job, was not in school and had no plans for the future. The other day, he received a letter from her:

> Dear Dad,
>
> This letter may be hard to take, so please sit down and have a cup of coffee while you read it.
>
> I know you don't like Bob, but if you would get to know him you'd like him as much as I do. I certainly hope so ... because I've decided to move in with Bob. It means I'll be further from the college, but that's something else I want to tell you ... I'm going to drop out of school and get a job to support us. I know how much you value education, but you also taught me to think for myself. And right now, that's what I think is best.
>
> Anyway, both Bob and I hope you'll take the time to get to know him because we've decided to get married. He's really great and I'm sure you'll like him when you get to know him.
>
> And the best news of all? I'm pregnant! So, I'm sure you'll agree our getting married is the best thing to do.
>
> Love,
> Your daughter, Amy

At the bottom of the page in small letters are the words, "Please turn over." Her father wondered what could possibly be next and quickly turned the page.

1

Dad,

I'm sorry to have put you through all that. I'm not pregnant and we're not getting married. I'm certainly not dropping out of school for Bob; I broke off with him a couple days ago. You were right, he was a jerk.

However, I did get a D in chemistry. I just wanted to put it in perspective.

This story makes an important point: Perspective is very important.

Much has been said, published and broadcast about America's health care system, the medical advances we have made and that it is the best health care system in the world. I would like to give you a different perspective.

Current Health Care Statistics

Cancer
According to the Centers for Disease Control and Prevention (CDC), the cancer rate in America more than doubled from the start of the War on Cancer in 1971 to the year 2001.[1] This was in spite of the fact that the National Cancer Institute's annual budget went from $150 million in 1971 to $4.6 billion in 2005, an increase of thirty times.[2] Now "40.77% of men and women born today will be diagnosed with cancer at some time during their lifetime"![3]

Heart Disease
One person in three suffers from some form of heart or circulatory system disease, including high blood pressure, heart disease and stroke. One out of every three people dies from these conditions. That

---

[1] Cancer Survivorship—United States, 1971–2001, Centers for Disease Control

[2] *Cancer-Gate: How to Win the Losing Cancer War*, Samuel S. Epstein, M.D., 2005

[3] National Cancer Institute statistics website, http://seer.cancer.gov/statfacts/html/all.html, accessed 6 Oct. 2010

is more than 2,400 deaths each day, an average of one death every 37 seconds.[4]

Diabetes
"The United States saw a 136 percent increase in the number of people with diabetes between 1980 and 2007."[5]

Obesity
The number of adults who are extremely obese and thus likely to have serious health problems increased 600% from 1961 to 2006, according to the CDC.[6] The extremely obese have more than twice the risk of heart disease, high blood pressure and diabetes than normal weight Americans.[7]

Cost of Health Care
Although America spent 36 times as much money as Cuba on health care in 1997 according to the World Health Organization ($3724 vs. $109), an American male was only expected to live one month longer than a Cuban male. Worse, a Cuban male could expect to remain healthy for one month longer at the end of his life than an American male. Even worse, the World Health Organization ranked Cuba's health level 36th in the world, while America's ranked 72nd out of 144.[8] By the way, who spent more than any other country in the world for health care? America.

These statistics clearly demonstrate there is something modern medicine does not know about these diseases that is important for their prevention. Why is this?

---

4 Presbyterian Hospital website, http://nyp.org/health/cardiac-stats.html, accessed 6 Oct. 2010

5 "Diabetes Epidemic Growing," CBS News website, Jun. 22, 2010, accessed 6 Oct. 2010

6 "Prevalence of overweight, obesity and extreme obesity among adults: United States, trends 1960-62 through 2005-2006," Centers for Disease Control and Prevention, Dec. 2008

7 "Health Implications of Obesity," National Institutes of Health Consensus Statement, Feb. 1985

8 *World Health Report 2000,* World Health Organization

Ideas in Conflict

Modern medicine is built on the concept of symptoms and disease. The modern medical doctor is taught to observe the patient's symptoms, run diagnostic tests and compare that information to symptoms of known diseases. After that process of diagnosis, he prescribes the currently accepted treatment to cure that disease and the patient hopefully gets well—meaning the patient no longer has those symptoms. This method may work well for infections, measles, etc. But heart disease, high blood pressure, obesity, diabetes, Alzheimer's and cancer are another matter, and a very serious one, because together they were the cause of death for more than half of all Americans who died in 2006, according to the CDC.

However, the medical disease concept is not the only concept of healing. There are others: chiropractic, acupuncture, traditional Chinese medicine and naturopathy. Naturopathic doctors teach their patients to use diet, exercise, lifestyle changes and natural therapies to enhance their bodies' ability to prevent and combat disease, according to the American Association of Naturopathic Physicians website. (Note the wording "doctors teach their patients ..." above. The word "doctor" actually comes from the Latin word docere, meaning to teach.) These alternative models of healing base their practices on the fact that the human body will heal itself if given the chance and the patient is taught how to do that. For example, when you cut yourself, the wound heals, provided you keep it clean and protected from being reopened again.

Diagnosis is not as important to these other schools of healing because it is recognized that if you give your body correct nutrition and exercise, detoxify it as needed, and eliminate negative mental influences and stress, the body will heal itself. This was the foundation of modern medicine as developed by Hippocrates, the Father of Medicine, 400 BC. However, medicine has not always stayed true to its roots.

Challenging Established Authority

Because other healing models accept other causes for lack of vibrant good health and happiness, they are often dismissed or even fought by medical societies. A historical example of this is Sir William A. Lane (1856–1943). He was a distinguished member of the British Royal Society of Surgeons. He is still known for three surgical procedures he

4

invented, including the use of plates and screws for repairing fractures that otherwise wouldn't heal correctly. During the First World War (1914–18), he opened a branch of Queen Mary's Hospital, which pioneered plastic surgery to repair facial birth defects.

"Lane was regarded at his peak as the best abdominal surgeon in England and was called on to operate on Royalty, politicians and many society figures of the Edwardian era."[9]

His vast experience in surgery led him to realize that long-term, uneliminated waste in the colon putrefied and therefore caused many other diseases. Lane referred to it as autointoxication (literally, self poisoning). The modern word for it is endotoxins (endo = internal, toxins = poisons). For example, such toxins are created when protein is acted on by certain bacteria. In his first misguided attempt to remedy this, Lane, being a surgeon, performed total colectomies (removing the entire colon).

In 1926, after observing the failure of surgery as a treatment for this condition, Lane "started promoting exercise, fruit and vegetables and bran cereal as the answer to bowel problems. Using his many royal and society connections, he set up the New Health Society [in England in 1925] to promote ... health education... [and] ... wrote columns in the newspapers, held public lectures and improved the distribution of fruit and vegetables."[10]

The medical establishment fought his effort to improve health with non-medicinal, non-surgical means. They were so vehement that in 1926, Lane, "in order to promote the New Health Society..., asked to have his name removed from the Medical Register to avoid being disciplined by the [British] General Medical Council."[11]

Addressing the Johns Hopkins Hospital and Medical College, Sir William A. Lane said:

9 "Sir William Arbuthnot-Lane," Wikipedia, the online encyclopedia, accessed, 6 Oct. 2010

10 Ibid.

11 Brand, Richard A. M.D., "Sir William Arbuthnot Lane, 1856–1943," Clinical Orthopedics [spine and joint medicine] and Related Research, Aug. 2009

"Gentlemen, I will never die of cancer. I am taking measures to prevent it... It is caused by poisons created in our bodies by the food we eat... What we should do, then, if we would avoid cancer, is to eat... raw fruits and vegetables; first, that we may be better nourished; secondly, that we may more easily eliminate waste products... We have been studying germs when we should have been studying diet and drainage... The world has been on the wrong track. The answer has been within ourselves all the time... Drain the body of its poisons, feed it properly, and the miracle is done. Nobody need have cancer who will take the trouble to avoid it."[12]

By the way, Lane lived to be 87 years old and died from being run over during the Second World War in London.[13]

Modern medicine does not classify "a growing lack of energy and enthusiasm toward life as you age" as a disease. So, if you experience this condition, do not expect a conventional doctor to be able to help you. Some even mislabel it, call it depression, and prescribe drugs with dangerous side effects. It is not that he does not care. It is that he has not been taught the name of a disease to match those symptoms and he does not have a drug or surgical operation to treat your condition. What other options are there?

Support for Alternative Medicine

Although modern medicine may have a poor view of it, fasting and severe calorie reduction is the only method proven to extend life uniformly for all members of a species and this has been proven in numerous scientific experiments since 1935. In that year, Dr. Clive McCay at Cornell University reported that rodents fed on a 30% reduced calorie diet increased their life span by 40%—that would be almost 30 more years for a human![14]

---

12 Malkmus, George, Rev., *Why Christians Get Sick*, Destiny Image Publishers, 2005

13 "Sir William Arbuthnot-Lane," Wikipedia, the online encyclopedia, accessed 6 Oct. 2010

14 "One for the Ages: A Prescription That May Extend Life," NY Times, Oct. 31, 2006

In addition to increased longevity, most age-related diseases, such as kidney degeneration or tumors, were also reduced. A later study published by the National Institutes of Health found monkeys on a 30% reduced calorie diet lived 15 years longer. And, like the rodents, the monkeys avoided much of the usual diseases of old age.[15]

Stephen R. Spindler, Ph.D., of the University of California Riverside, has proven in his experiments that calorie restriction partially restored liver function in mice and reduced inflammation.[16]

Allan Cott, M.D. was no stranger to the benefits of fasting. He wrote the 1975 bestselling book, *Fasting — The Ultimate Diet*.[17] The cover of his book quotes the *New England Journal of Medicine* as saying, "Fasting is a valid experience. It can benefit any otherwise healthy person whose calories now have the upper hand in his/her life." His book cites 329 references on fasting: 158 are scientific or medical journals. In his 1977 book, *Fasting as a Way of Life*, Cott includes an entire chapter on the resistance shown by many in modern medicine who have not actually had any first- or second-hand experience.[18]

Dr. Cott, a psychiatrist, got interested in fasting when he learned that the Russian psychiatrist Dr. Yuri Nikolayev had successfully treated 7,000 neurotic, psychotic and schizophrenic patients with fasting alone after they had not been helped by drugs or other means.[19]

Carlos Garcia, M.D. and Elson Haas, M.D. are two contemporary examples of medical doctors who have discovered more natural ways to help the body heal itself. More are doing this every day.

America's Health Care Crisis

Much has been said in health care reform about the millions of Americans not covered by health insurance. The mistaken assumption is that our current health care system just needs to be expanded to give more people access to doctors, drugs and hospitals. More money, more drugs and more days in the hospital are not necessarily the answer

---

15 Ibid.

16 "Proceedings of the National Academy of Sciences," Dec. 2001

17 Cott, Alan, *Fasting—The Ultimate Diet*, Hastings House, 1975

18 Cott, Alan, *Fasting as a Way of Life*, Hastings House, 1977

19 Ibid.

to better health. If you doubt that, reread the comparison of Cuban health with American health above.

Your health is your responsibility. Learn what works for your body. Consult with health care experts, do your own research, but you choose what to believe and act on.

Part II:

Anti-Aging

The current word for looking and feeling younger is "anti-aging," which can mean different things to different people. Women in their thirties and forties use it to mean looking younger, and having less wrinkles and lines. Fifty- and sixty-year-olds frequently use it to mean being free of the diseases of old age: heart disease, cancer, diabetes, high blood pressure, Alzheimer's and arthritis. Other people in their fifties, sixties and seventies think of it as extending life. Happily, they are all related. The following studies will show you that when you successfully extend life, you also reduce the risk for the diseases of old age, and you look younger!

Scientific Studies

There has only been one scientifically proven method of extending life beyond the normal span of years, demonstrated over and over in eight different species of life, from single-celled yeast to monkeys.[1] (The studies on man are mentioned below.) This method is calorie restriction, which consists of reducing the amount of calories consumed by 30% to 40%, while ensuring optimum nutrition. This method was originally shown in 1934 to nearly double the life span of laboratory rats.[2]

Some would argue that it has been known for thousands of years.

One-quarter of what you eat keeps you alive.

The other three-quarters keeps your doctor alive.

Hieroglyph found in an ancient Egyptian tomb

---

1 "Calorie Restriction," Wikipedia, the online encyclopedia, accessed 12 Oct. 2010

2 "Prolonging the Life Span," *The Scientific Monthly*, 1934

The above Egyptian hieroglyph would be a fitting summary for a twenty-year study on monkeys begun in 1989. It showed that monkeys on calorie restriction lived longer *with less age-related diseases* (heart disease, diabetes, cancer and brain degeneration) *and looked younger* than monkeys free to eat all they wanted. Among the animals eating all they wanted, 13% developed diabetes and 29% became pre-diabetic. *None* of the calorie-restricted animals showed any such problems. The monkeys eating all they wanted had twice the rate of cancer, twice the rate of heart disease and three times the rate of diabetes and/or arthritis.[3]

You may wonder, "Why not study humans?" A study of humans would have to run at least eighty years to *prove* life extension. Fortunately, there have been "short" human studies that show the same kind of improvements in health. One six-month study reported a significantly lower risk of diabetes and reduced DNA damage.[4] (DNA is the chemical that controls how new cells are created. Less DNA damage means less abnormal cells and increased cellular health.) Another human study showed dramatic, long-term reduction in major heart disease factors "that usually increase with advancing age."[5] The calorie-restricted group (ages 35–82) had triglyceride (blood fat) levels equal to the very healthiest twenty-year-olds, and their blood pressure levels were the equivalent of ten-year-old children!

Other wise men have known this for hundreds of years:

"To lengthen thy Life, lessen thy meals."
Benjamin Franklin

---

3 "Caloric restriction delays disease onset and mortality in rhesus monkeys," *Science*, 2009

4 "Effect of 6-Month Calorie Restriction on Biomarkers of Longevity, Metabolic Adaptation, and Oxidative Stress in Overweight Individuals," *Journal of the American Medical Assn.*, 2006

5 "Long-term calorie restriction is highly effective in reducing the risk for atherosclerosis in humans," *Proceedings of the National Academy of Sciences*, 2004

A More Practical Approach

There are two methods of calorie reduction: continuous and intermittent (on and off). A frequent drawback to continuous calorie restriction is hunger. Another drawback is social occasions. Both of these make calorie restriction difficult. So, intermittent calorie restriction gives the advantage that you can eat anything you want the next day, making it easier.

One study of intermittent calorie reduction found that over a year, mice fed three weeks on and three weeks off a 50% restricted diet with optimum nutrition had eight times less tumors than mice that ate all they wanted![6] More relevantly, a study of humans who fasted one day a month showed they were 39% less likely to have heart disease.[7]

Fasting for more than three days, however, has the advantage that after the first two or three days hunger generally disappears, and fasting as a means of calorie restriction offers the same health benefits.

One hundred seventy-four people with high blood pressure were treated with a water-only fast for ten to eleven days under medical supervision, and then approximately six days on a low-fat, low-salt, vegan diet. All those who were on medication for high blood pressure were able to discontinue their medication after this treatment.[8]

This last study was repeated a year later on sixty-eight patients with borderline high blood pressure.[9] (Borderline high blood pressure is higher than normal, but not so alarming that medications are immediately essential.) This study also found that water-only fasting reduced blood pressure in the overwhelming majority of cases. More interesting, however, was the finding that drug treatment for high blood pressure on average only lowered it by twelve points; a low-sodium, low-fat,

---

6 "Serum Insulin-like Growth Factor-I and Mammary Tumor Development in Ad libitum-Fed, Chronic Calorie-Restricted, and Intermittent Calorie-Restricted MMTV-TGF-α Mice," *Cancer Prevention Research*, Aug. 2009

7 "Occasional Fasting Associated With Lower Heart Disease Rates." *ScienceDaily*, Nov. 2007 accessed 17 Oct. 2010

8 "Medically supervised water-only fasting in the treatment of hypertension," *Journal of Manipulative Physiological Therapeutics*, 2001

9 "Medically supervised water-only fasting in the treatment of borderline hypertension," *Journal of Alternative and Complementary Medicine*, 2002

vegan diet with exercise on average lowered it by sixteen points; and the previous water-only fasting study showed it was lowered by thirty-nine points! Perhaps natural treatment *is* better.

An interesting measure of rejuvenation not mentioned by modern researchers is sexual potency, fertility and drive. Although modern researchers have not mentioned it, it is well documented in the work of Herbert Shelton, who used fasting to treat 35,000 patients at his Natural Hygiene School.[10] He says in *The Science and Fine Art of Fasting* that although it is not a hard and fast rule, sexual desire and potency usually disappear during the fast and return at the end of it.[11] Then he cites several cases of men and women who regained potency and fertility as a result of the fast. (By the way, I have received emails from two women who were unable to conceive before the Master Cleanse, who conceived within a few months of completing it.)

There is another experiment in life extension that is seldom mentioned, but it reveals another reason that calorie restriction works to extend life. Besides, it is a great story.

The Chicken Heart that Lived Forever

On January 17, 1912, a Nobel-prize-winning surgeon, Alexis Carrel, extracted a tiny piece of heart muscle from a chicken embryo and placed it in fresh nutrient solution. In order to remove the metabolic wastes constantly being generated by it, every forty-eight hours he would transfer it to a new flask with a fresh, clean bath of nutrients. Because it grew, the heart muscle had to be regularly trimmed before being moved to its next flask. Thirty years later the tissue was still growing! Keep in mind that the average chicken lives for five to seven years, twenty years being the longest.

When Carrel died in 1944, the tissue was still living. It continued to live until April 1946, when the experiment was deliberately ended.[12]

---

10 Shelton, Herbert M., *The Science and Fine Art of Fasting*, Natural Hygiene Press, Chicago, IL, 1978, p. 66

11 Ibid., pp. 163-168

12 "Alexis Carrel—Biography," http://www.alenasites.com/alexis-carrel/ accessed 20 Oct. 2010

Anti-Aging

Later scientists have not been able to repeat this experiment with the same results, but no one argues that the chicken heart lived for thirty-four years.

This experiment points out the importance of eliminating metabolic wastes, which are by-products of digestion and other normal body functions. They are toxic and must be eliminated; for example, digestion of animal protein produces uric acid which must be eliminated in the urine. Shelton even gives laboratory reports of the amount of toxins eliminated on fasts in *The Science and Fine Art of Fasting*.[13]

I have heard people say there is no need for cleansing because the body's elimination systems normally handle that. That may be true for someone who always exercises, drinks plenty of water, eats plenty of vegetables every day and never smokes, drinks, eats junk food nor over-eats. However, I have never met such a person.

Most people have a backlog of waste that the body's elimination systems will handle *if given the chance*. Giving it that chance means a regular period of restricting the quantity and type of food (no junk food, for instance), and can include water fasting, juice fasting or living on a restricted diet of healthy food only.

My Experience with the Master Cleanse

I always feel younger when I am on the Master Cleanse and I frequently hear from people doing the Master Cleanse that their friends say they look ten years younger. A few years ago while I was on the Master Cleanse, I took my grandson, who was probably seven at the time, to the park and we played tag. I was running all around and having a good time. Two somewhat older children watched us for a while and then joined us in the game and we all had a good time. Afterward, my grandson said something to me and called me by his nickname for me, "Pepa," pronounced "Pee-Pa." The other boys asked what that was and I told them it meant "Grandfather." They refused to believe it. They said grandparents just do not run around and play tag. I guess their grandparents did not know about the Master Cleanse.

---

13 Shelton, Herbert M., *The Science and Fine Art of Fasting*, Natural Hygiene Press, Chicago, IL, 1978, pp.151-154

My point is that the Master Cleanse done three or four times a year as recommended by Stanley Burroughs, the developer of the Master Cleanse, acts as intermittent fasting. In between cleanses, he recommends a vegetarian diet that excludes meat, dairy, fish and processed foods.[14] Such a diet, especially one that includes lots of green leafy vegetables, would resupply the body with the alkaline minerals necessary to neutralize the acidic toxins that are first mobilized from the fat cells and connective tissue, then neutralized in the liver and finally eliminated.

What About Protein, Vitamins and Minerals?

Allan Cott, M.D., wrote a million-copy, bestselling book in 1975 called *Fasting: The Ultimate Diet*. He followed it two years later with *Fasting as a Way of Life*. Because of the feedback he had received from his first book, he wrote, "If disparaging doctors would take the time to examine the evidence [...], they would finally stop warning of 'dangers' that simply do not exist for most people."[15]

The average person has enough nutritional reserves of all kinds to fast (water only) for at least a month.[16,17,18,19,20] So, doing a Master Cleanse for ten days or more is no problem for most people.

---

14 Burroughs, Stanley, *The Master Cleanser*, Burroughs Books, Reno, NV, 1976, p.27

15 Cott, Allan, M.D., *Fasting as a Way of Life*, Hastings House, Norwalk, CT, 1977, p. 2

16 Fuhrman, Joel, M.D., *Fasting and Eating for Health*, St. Martin's Griffin, New York, NY, p. 13

17 Anton J. Carlson, Prof. of Physiology at the University of Chicago, as quoted on by Herbert Shelton in *The Science and Fine Art of Fasting*, p. 66

18 Burroughs, Stanley, *The Master Cleanser*, Burroughs Books, Reno, NV, 1976

19 Cott, Allan, M.D., *Fasting: The Ultimate Diet*, Hastings House, Norwalk, CT, 1975, p. 57

20 McCoy, Frank, M.D., *The Fast Way to Health*, 11th ed., originally published in 1926, published as an eBook by Peter Glickman, Inc., 2009, p. 20

The need for protein is *greatly* exaggerated in our society. How many people do you know personally with the following symptoms of protein deficiency: apathy, a swollen belly (not fat, just swollen), swollen legs, stunted growth, flaky skin and mental retardation? Have you seen many people around you that have those symptoms?

More likely, you have seen people with mental fogginess, headaches, dehydration, and a higher risk of osteoporosis, heart disease and cancer. Would you be surprised to learn those are the symptoms of too much protein?

The Future

Thomas Edison was a remarkable man. He imagined recording a performance and being able to hear it again later. Then he invented the phonograph. He imagined being able to create light in the darkness. Then he invented the electric light and all the other necessary items to provide electricity to cities. He imagined being able to record pictures that moved. Then he invented the motion picture camera. Edison observed the medical system of his day, drawing the following conclusion (as reported in articles from late 1902 and early 1903[21]):

"The doctor of the future will give no medicine, but will instruct his patient in the care of the human frame, in diet and in the cause and prevention of disease."
Thomas Edison

The future is here. Use what you know about nutrition to extend your life and health.

21 http://www.snopes.com/quotes/edison.asp accessed Oct.25, 2010

Part III:

How to Do the Master Cleanse

Shopping List

IMPORTANT NOTE: These quantities are based on six glasses of lemonade per day for the minimum of ten days. You should drink six to twelve glasses of lemonade per day. So, you may have to multiply these quantities if you drink more glasses per day or go longer than ten days.

- Books: *Lose Weight, Have More Energy & Be Happier in 10 Days* by Peter Glickman and/or *The Master Cleanser* by Stanley Burroughs

- 30 large lemons, 60 limes or small lemons, or a combination. Only buy half this amount and the other half later, if you buy organic, which is preferred. Organic spoils faster than conventional fruit.

- 64 fluid ounces organic Grade B maple syrup or the darkest organic maple syrup you can find

- At least four ounces of sea salt that does not say "iodized" or "iodine added"

- At least six teaspoons (about one half ounce) of cayenne pepper powder, not capsules. Regular cayenne is about 30,000 heat units. You can use hotter if you like.

- A box of at least ten herbal laxative tea bags. I recommend those teas with 50 percent senna rather than pure senna leaf tea.

- At least eight gallons of spring, purified or distilled water without added fluoride or chlorine for the lemonade, salt water flush and a cup of laxative tea each evening. Fluoride was used for decades as rat poison. It is very injurious to human health and studies have shown it to increase the risk of cancer and hip fractures.

- One box or bottle of probiotics to be taken per the directions on the bottle or box after you return to eating solid food.

- These ingredients should be easy to find at any health food store, not grocery store. If you cannot find these easily, you can order them either at **www.TheMasterCleanse.com**/store, or if you have Peter Glickman's Master Cleanse Coach iPhone app, use the Supplies link on the first or second page.

- Do not buy cayenne in capsules. According to Dr. Richard Schulze, a master herbalist, people who take cayenne capsules do not receive much of the benefit of the cayenne. The nerve endings in the mouth respond almost instantly to send blood throughout the body. This whole process is missed if you take capsules. People who "hate" it or "can't stand it" have simply used too much for their first taste. It is a learned taste. The way to handle "hating" it is to start by adding only a sprinkle and then gradually build up the amount as you can tolerate it.

- Do not buy pre-mixed powders or ingredients. They must be pasteurized by law, which kills most of the enzymes in the lemon/lime juice. I know from the personal experience of coaching someone who was using bottled lemon juice that it did not produce very good results until she switched to fresh squeezed lemon juice. Likewise, avoid all powders and pills for the same reason: dehydrated powders do not have the same effectiveness as fresh enzymes.

- Do not buy additional vitamins or supplements. Burroughs says three times in his book, The Master Cleanser, not to take any other supplements. Fasting has been a powerful and natural way to heal and rejuvenate the body for thousands of years. Animals instinctively fast when they are ill. The Master Cleanse is a juice fast. Adding anything to it merely reduces the power of the fast.

- Do not buy kits that contain less than 64 ounces of organic maple syrup. Some providers try to lower their price by shorting the amount of maple syrup because maple syrup is the most expensive item in the cleanse.

Quick Start

They say you cannot please everyone, but I am going to try. There are those people who like to have all the information before they start. I understand you because I am like that most of the time. However, sometimes I just want to jump in and start. If I need the details, I will get them when I need them. For you, I have created this Quick Start.

Just begin here and consult the index or alphabetical table of contents for whatever details you need when you need them.

Read the Shopping List before this section, if you have not already done so.

- The night before and every night of the cleanse, drink one cup of herbal laxative tea before bed.

- Before drinking any lemonade, each day of the cleanse, drink thirty-two ounces of spring, purified or distilled water with two TEASPOONS of sea salt.

- During each day of the cleanse, drink 6 to 12 glasses of lemonade:

    2 tablespoons (1 fluid ounce) of fresh-squeezed lemon/lime juice

    2 tablespoons (1 fluid ounce) of organic, Grade B maple syrup

    1/10 teaspoon of cayenne pepper or to taste

    8 ounce of medium-hot (or cold if you prefer) spring, purified or distilled water.

- As much herbal mint tea and/or water as you wish.

- Do not eat anything else; no solid food. The only exception is prescribed medications. Do not discontinue prescriptions without consulting a licensed health care practitioner.

- Breaking the cleanse: First day after the cleanse, slowly drink several glasses of freshly squeezed orange juice. If you experience any digestive problems, dilute the orange juice with water. Second day, freshly squeezed orange juice all day for vegetarians. Others should make a homemade vegetable soup in the afternoon from several different vegetables, such as carrots, celery, potatoes, onions, tomatoes, green peppers, zucchini, beans, peas, lentils, brown rice, and dehydrated veggies or spices. Use sea salt sparingly. No meat or meat stock. Drink mostly the broth for dinner. Third day, freshly squeezed orange juice in the morning for vegetarians, followed by fresh fruit for lunch and a fruit or raw vegetable salad for dinner. Others drink orange juice in the morning, have the rest of the soup for lunch and eat a vegetarian dinner limited to fruit, salad or vegetables.

- I recommend on the third day after the cleanse, you begin to take probiotics per the instructions on the box or bottle to replace any good bacteria that may have been flushed out of you.

More Details

1. Length of Time, and Frequency

The Master Cleanse should be done for at least ten days. Burroughs says it can be done for forty or more days. I've personally done it more than nine times from ten to twenty-eight days (and once for three days) —all within two years. Burroughs is right about ten days being the minimum. The three-day Master Cleanse left me feeling as though nothing had been accomplished. I can hear you saying, "Ten days?! Is he crazy?" Amazingly, you will not be hungry and you will have more energy than you felt before the Master Cleanse.

In addition to my own longer Master Cleanses, I know of three other people who have done it for twenty days. All of us found that there were spiritual gains after eight or ten days: a clarity of purpose, a sense of focus, a feeling of well being, and a discovery that our natural emotion is one of cheerful satisfaction.

Burroughs says the best sign that the Master Cleanse is complete is a clear, pink tongue. Your tongue will definitely get coated and turn white and possibly other colors. Not everyone continues until their tongue is clear and pink. If you want to quit sooner, you can. The Master Cleanse is not like a school grade that you only do once. You can do it three or four times a year, each time detoxing more. Most stop at ten days regardless of tongue color. However, ten days is long enough to make a major change in your weight, health and mental outlook.

How soon can you do another Master Cleanse? It's best to space out your Master Cleanses by three or four months and eat lots of fresh greens and salads in between or drink daily green smoothies. You need to build up your calcium, magnesium and potassium reserves because the body uses those alkaline minerals to neutralize the toxins before they are eliminated. Very rarely (three out of a thousand), a person has done a Master Cleanse every month for several months in a row, which resulted in temporary hair loss. It was handled by taking lots of vitamins and minerals, but it is better to avoid that.

Refined sugar reduces calcium in the bones and teeth as the body needs to balance the blood chemistry after eating sugar, and it uses calcium to do that, which it will pull from the teeth and bones if there is no alkaline mineral reserve. Perhaps the epidemic of osteoporosis is no more than the popularity of a diet with too much sugar and not enough fresh, raw greens! By the way, milk is not a good source of calcium for building reserves. It is too hard for most people to digest it.

2. Laxative Tea

Drink one cup of herbal laxative tea before bed on the night before and every night thereafter while you are on the cleanse, unless you have diarrhea. (Diarrhea is NOT watery eliminations within two hours of drinking the salt water flush.) If you have diarrhea, discontinue the laxative tea and salt water flush until it stops. You can buy herbal laxative tea in most health food stores. There are two types I am aware of: pure senna tea and combinations of senna with other herbs. I recommend herbal laxative bags with 50 percent senna leaf rather than pure senna leaf tea. Senna is a powerful laxative and too much may cause cramps, particularly in the later days of a cleanse when there is little in the intestines. Although not painful, they are uncomfortable and can cause unnecessary concern. If such cramps do occur, they can be turned off quite quickly by drinking water or lemonade.

I personally did not have any problem with senna until my third Master Cleanse. Then I felt uncomfortably strong contractions and switched to a combination tea. Occasionally, when I run out of the combination, I'll make half a cup and dilute it. Such a combination tea is Get Regular from Yogi Teas.

I have been asked (rarely) if senna is addictive or will cause damage. I have never seen or heard of damage or addiction with any of the thousands of people who have done the Master Cleanse of whom I am aware. Perhaps 10 percent have reported uncomfortable cramps. In my experience, the cramps have disappeared when the salt water or lemonade is drunk and can be avoided by using the combination teas. The senna box warns not to give it to children or to drink more than two cups per day. The combination box says not to drink more than four cups per day and half that for children from six to twelve years old.

3. Salt Water Flush

Before drinking any lemonade, each day of the cleanse, drink a quart of water with two teaspoons of non-iodized sea salt. Drink it all at once or as close to that as you can. Non-iodized sea salt is sea salt that does not say "Iodine added" or "Iodized." It is easier to drink than bleached pure white table salt. The other reason to use non-iodized sea salt is that it contains vital trace minerals that your body needs. Non-iodized sea salt does not mean no iodine. It means no additional iodine has been added. Any brand will do. I personally recommend Light Grey Celtic Sea Salt, which can be found at most health food stores. Do not drink any lemonade or take any prescribed medications for a half hour after drinking the salt water.

This should produce several urgent and intense eliminations within an hour. If it does not, gradually increase the amount of sea salt. If that does not work, try a little less sea salt. These urgent eliminations generally take place for forty-five to sixty minutes. Plan two hours before you leave the house after drinking the salt water flush. After a couple days of salt water flushes, you can gauge how much time you need, but two hours is generally safe.

Some people have trouble with drinking the salt water. Be sure you stir the salt water so the salt is evenly distributed in the drink just before you drink it. It will be easier to drink and it is more effective. I believe it is very important to include it. So try everything you can. My wife found it helpful to drink it through a straw or to count the number of swallows as you drink it. Do not add anything to the salt water to make it taste better. Stay with the program. If you find that you absolutely cannot drink the salt water, Burroughs says you can drink another cup of herbal laxative tea in the morning instead. However, the laxative stimulates the muscles of the intestinal wall to contract and mechanically move the waste through. The salt water flushes whatever loose waste is in the digestive tract and the salt also helps to dissolve the mucus and waste.

Many people have noticed that it is much easier to drink the salt water flush on later days of a cleanse. I believe this may be because the body reacts more dramatically when it has more mucus in the system and, as that gets cleaned out, the body has less reaction to the salt water flush.

The reason for two teaspoons of salt is to increase the weight (specific gravity) of the salt water until it matches the weight of blood. Specific gravity is how heavy the substance is compared to an equal volume of water. When the salt water and the blood are the same weight, the body will treat the salt water as though it were blood, not absorb the salt from the digestive system, and will just "flush" the salt water through the system instead of absorbing it.

● People who have recently been on the Atkins diet or any heavy meat and dairy diet may need two or three days before the flush produces eliminations. This is because meat and dairy are frequently hard to digest and build up waste that clogs the colon.

After the Master Cleanse, you may do the salt water flush whenever you want to clean your intestines. Just be sure to do it on an empty stomach.

4. The Drink: Lemons, Maple Syrup, Cayenne, Water

If you drink less than six glasses a day, you will not lose as much weight and may have more severe detox symptoms. Here are the recipes:

Ideal recipe, if freshly extracted sugar cane juice is available:

- 10 ounces of medium-hot or cold, freshly extracted sugar cane juice

- 2 tablespoons (1 fluid ounce) of fresh squeezed lemon/lime juice

- 1/10 teaspoon of cayenne pepper or to taste

Next best recipe:

- 2 tablespoons (1 fluid ounce) of freshly squeezed lemon/lime juice

- 2 tablespoons (1 fluid ounce) of organic Grade B maple syrup

- 1/10 teaspoon of cayenne pepper or to taste

- 8 ounces of medium-hot (or cold if you prefer) spring, purified or distilled water

The enzymes in the lemon break down the layers of old waste in the colon. Although the lemon is acidic, it becomes alkaline when digested and the alkalinity helps neutralize the acidity of the toxic wastes. Try to get organic lemons from your local health food store, if possible, as they contain more minerals than non-organic ones. The lemon juice must be fresh squeezed, not bottled. The enzymes begin to break down within hours and heating (Pasteurizing) kills them completely. If you must prepare the drinks for most of the day—for taking to work, for example—prepare only that much and make fresh lemonade when you get home for the rest of the day. To make up more than one day's lemonade at one time or to try to save the squeezed lemon juice for another day will lose a great deal of the potency of the lemons.

Burroughs says to never to vary the amount of lemon juice in each drink. You can increase or decrease the maple syrup, but not the amount of the lemon juice.

The maple syrup supplies the sugar for energy and more importantly, it supplies the needed minerals. Use the darkest organic maple syrup you can find, which in the U.S. is Grade B. A is lighter than B. The darker the syrup, the more minerals. So try to get B if possible, but any organic grade will do. There is no Grade C anymore. If you are buying Canadian syrup, just get the darkest organic maple syrup you can find. The reason for organic is that some companies use formaldehyde in the process of tapping the trees. Organic grade B maple syrup can be found in most health food stores.

If you cannot find maple syrup, freshly extracted sugar cane juice makes the ideal lemonade drink. See the previous page for the recipe. A less-than-optimum substitute is sorghum, but Burroughs says it does not produce results as good. Use two tablespoons, the same amount as maple syrup.

If you are diabetic see the section "For Those With Diabetes or High Blood Pressure" below.

Agave nector should not be used. Agave must be heated to make it sweet. The heating creates fructose and agave has more fructose than high fructose corn syrup, which was linked to obesity in a Princeton University study.[1]

Cayenne pepper contains Vitamin A, several B vitamins and Vitamin C and has been used by master herbalists for dilating blood vessels, dissolving mucus and feeding the heart. It is sold in several heat strengths as measured in heat units. If you do not usually eat hot food, buy the 30,000 heat unit cayenne. African Bird Pepper is 80,000 heat units. It is really hot.

I know I am repeating myself, but this is important. If you do not like cayenne pepper, you may be tempted to take capsules, leave it out

---

1   "High-fructose corn syrup causes characteristics of obesity in rats: increased body weight, body fat and triglyceride levels," Bocarsly ME, Powell ES, Avena NM, Hoebel BG., *Pharmacology, biochemistry, and behavior*, Nov. 2010

or take a concentrated dose and then drink the lemonade without the pepper. Do not do these things. Cayenne acts like an accelerator pedal for the cleanse. It is a learned taste, meaning you have to try it a few times before you like it. So, if you do not like it, just add a tiny pinch to the first few drinks and gradually build up the amount as it is comfortable for you to do.

Another reason not to take cayenne in capsules is the body must digest the capsule to gain the benefit of the cayenne. You are not eating anything that requires digestion to give your digestive system a chance to rest as well as cleanse itself. Since digestion uses 30 percent of the body's energy, you are gaining more usable energy by eliminating digestion. So, taking cayenne capsules should not be done.

5. Water/Mint Tea

In addition to the above, you may drink as much spring, distilled or purified water as you wish and occasionally some mint tea for a change. Do not use fluoridated water.

6. No Other Food or Drink

Nothing else is eaten or drunk on the Master Cleanse.

7. Breaking the Master Cleanse

Breaking the Master Cleanse diet correctly is very important! I have heard one second-hand story of someone coming off a long water fast, then going straight to overeating ribs and dessert, who then had serious medical problems. I do not know if this story is true, but I know personally that diving immediately back into a bad diet will make you feel very sick for a few hours. Correctly breaking the Master Cleanse is VERY important. I did it wrong once and had nausea and stomach pains for more than an hour. The longer your Master Cleanse is, the more important is how you break it.

I advise that you take one box or bottle of probiotics (following the directions on the bottle or box) after every cleanse to replace the good bacteria in your intestines that was eliminated on the cleanse. I discovered this after my third cleanse when I suddenly had intense cravings for "bad" food and taking probiotics eliminated the cravings for me. Probiotics make up 30 percent of the volume of your solid eliminations and so help to bring you back to regularity after the cleanse. They also produce vitamins A, B1, B2, B3, B12, and K; kill some of the disease-causing germs in your intestines; prevent bad bacteria (the bacteria that cause candida, for example) from getting out of control; and—some recent studies report—lower cholesterol and help in cases of irritable bowel syndrome (diarrhea, pain, and heightened food sensitivities). Antibiotics, while they are good for curing infections, destroy both good and bad bacteria. People, after taking antibiotics, should take probiotics to re-establish the good bacteria so necessary to health

If you usually eat meat, Burroughs says to break the fast slowly by drinking several glasses of orange juice for the first day and through the afternoon of the second. You may dilute the juice if you like or if you have any digestive problems. For dinner on the second day, drink mostly the broth of a homemade vegetable soup you make that afternoon from several different vegetables, beans and grains, such as carrots, celery, potatoes, onions, tomatoes, green peppers, zucchini, beans, peas, lentils, etc. No meat or meat stock. You may add brown rice and dehydrated veggies or spices, but use sea salt sparingly. The less you cook the soup, the better. You may have rye wafers with the soup, but not bread or crackers. Make enough for lunch the next day.

On the third day, drink orange juice in the morning. Have the rest of the soup for lunch. For dinner, eat whatever vegetarian salads, vegetables or fruit you wish. Begin eating your usual food the fourth day, although Burroughs recommends lemonade or fruit juice for breakfast on a continuing basis and a vegetarian diet as the best means of preserving life-long health.

If you are a vegetarian, drink fresh orange juice the first, second and morning of the third day. For lunch on the third day have raw fruit, with a raw fruit or vegetable salad for dinner. After that, eat normally. I used to find the orange juice too rich for me and chose to drink grapefruit juice instead when coming off the Master Cleanse.

If you have gas or digestive upset when breaking the fast, continue the Master Cleanse a few more days.

● For Those With Diabetes or High Blood Pressure

I have seen the Master Cleanse work very well for diabetics and I have heard of a case where it did not appear to work for a person. So, I am faithfully passing along Stanley Burroughs' instructions for diabetics as written in his book, Healing for the Age of Enlightenment. If you are a diabetic and wish to do the Master Cleanse, regularly test your blood sugar levels and do it in consulation with a licensed health care practitioner.

To start:

- 2 tablespoons (1 fluid ounce) of freshly squeezed lemon or lime juice

- Barely 1 tablespoon of molasses

- 1/10 teaspoon of cayenne pepper or to taste

- 8 ounces of medium-hot (or cold if you prefer) spring, purified or distilled water

- On following days, gradually increase the molasses by fractions of a tablespoon while monitoring blood sugar and reducing insulin. When 2 tablespoons of molasses have been achieved, check to see if it's possible to eliminate the insulin. Then use 2 tablespoons of maple syrup per drink.

You may drink as much herbal mint tea and/or water as you wish, providing that you drink at least six lemonades per day.

If you are on medication for high blood pressure, be aware that the Master Cleanse lowers most people's blood pressure. It is well documented in scientific literature that fasting lowers blood pressure.[2] This means if you are on medication for high blood pressure you will need to coordinate with a licensed health care practitioner as it is extremely likely that your blood pressure will come down. Likewise, when standing up from a sitting or lying position, do so slowly as you may feel dizzy.

If you are on anti-depression medication, consult with your prescribing health care practitioner. Some medications require food, others may require a lower dose while fasting. If you are interested in coming off these medications, visit www.TheRoadBack.org. But do not combine their program with the Master Cleanse. Do their program, then the Master Cleanse.

Detox Symptoms—the Good, the Bad and the Ugly

Detox symptoms are what you feel when toxins are mobilized, but not yet eliminated. Although detoxification symptoms are unpleasant, they ought to be desired. No one wants the feelings associated with detoxifying, but that is the purpose of the cleanse. If you are not

---

2 "Medically supervised water-only fasting in the treatment of hypertension," *Journal of Manipulative Physiological Therapeutics*, 2001

detoxifying, you are not making progress and will not feel better afterward!

I place detox symptoms into five classes. Knowing these symptoms will be gone in a day or two, it is much easier to persevere and complete the cleanse.

1. Cravings. I have noticed I crave things for a few hours or a day. Usually after the next morning's elimination, the craving is gone and I feel better. As your body detoxifies (eliminates the toxic waste from) cooked meat, dairy products, etc., it craves the hamburger, pizza, ice cream, etc. that is being "peeled off" in layers. Paavo Airola discusses this concept on page 153 of his book How to Get Well. If you think about it, smokers who quit are immediately subject to intense cravings for the same toxins their bodies are eliminating now that they have been given the chance. The same thing is true of drug addicts.

   This is why Burroughs says addicts can more easily quit their habits while on the Master Cleanse. It helps reduce the cravings that are the largest barrier to quitting.

2. Tiredness. It should not be strange that deleted toxins which age you and drain your energy should make you tired. When your body fights toxins, whether from detoxifying or from an infection, it diverts energy into healing and away from the energy you use to work and play. Toxins only make you tired until they are eliminated. That is why both the herbal laxative tea and salt water flush are so important. They are the "Agitator" and "Rinse Cycle" of the Master Cleanse. Most people have a day or two when they feel tired. Give yourself permission to rest on those days.

3. Irritability, boredom, etc. The irritability of dieters is common knowledge. Among the reasons for this is that reduced eating allows the body to detoxify and one of the symptoms of detoxification is irritability. In this class of symptoms, I also include boredom, anxiety, wanting to "just chew something," and wanting to quit the Master Cleanse. It is quite remarkable how the next day's eliminations can change your attitude toward the Master Cleanse.

   When you get to Day 8 or so, you may discover for yourself that your natural mood is positive and cheerful. I have a friend in Georgia who told me how surprised he was that he was able to stay so upbeat during the Master Cleanse in the face of some serious problems.

4.   Physical aches, pains, nausea, vomiting, etc. A few people on the Master Cleanse get headaches or other aches, in my experience perhaps 5 percent or less.

●   Those who get headaches usually had a caffeine habit (coffee or soft drinks) before starting on the Master Cleanse. Detoxifying from caffeine with the Master Cleanse with the salt water flush and laxative tea is probably much easier than going off it "cold turkey." Caffeine headaches are usually one or two days. The longest I have heard was four days. Persist. Nausea and vomiting are much rarer, but not unheard of. Again these are detox symptoms and will go away.

Other people may have aches and pains from previous illnesses for a few days before these aches and pains disappear a few days later. A friend had very severe hemorrhoids prior to the Master Cleanse. They appeared a few days after he started and went away a few days later. It was his impression that they would not be back.

5.   Hot or burning bowel movements. Toxins and other waste are acidic. I have found that when I eliminate old waste and other toxins, my bowel movements are actually hot. During my first Master Cleanse, my eliminations actually burned. I have also noticed that when I have serious detox symptoms as listed above, my eliminations the next morning are typically hot. This may be so bad in the first few days that you need to put some Vitamin E oil on your butt to soothe it. It acts within minutes.

Occasionally, someone will ask if it is the cayenne that burns. While cayenne in large quantities can temporarily cause hot bowel movements, this does not explain how—on a constant dose of cayenne—one can suddenly experience hot bowel movements after several days of normal temperatures. No, I am convinced it is the acidic toxins being eliminated.

In medicine, these detox symptoms are called Herxheimer Reactions. In alternative medicine, they are also called healing crises. They are a double-edged sword. Detox symptoms are a milestone in the detoxifying process indicating you are mobilizing and eliminating toxins. Unfortunately, they do not make you feel good.

It is important for someone on the Master Cleanse to know what detox symptoms are and that they usually will go away or be reduced with the next morning's eliminations. The exceptions are headaches due to caffeine withdrawal during the first few days, which may last two to four days, and rashes, which indicate a significant detoxification and may continue for several days. It is next to impossible to go ten consecutive days of cravings or tiredness with no relief in sight, but when you know those feelings will be gone with tomorrow's eliminations, anyone can make it through the Master Cleanse. The Master Cleanse is not about will power. It is about knowledge—what to expect and how to deal with it.

If you had severe symptoms, you might want to consider putting yourself on a health-restoring regimen for several months. Such a regimen should include:

1) Not filling the body with more toxins such as: refined white flour and sugar products, meat, artificial flavors, colors, preservatives, alcohol, tobacco, dairy products, etc.

2) Detoxifying the colon to eliminate the toxins being reabsorbed by the blood and redistributed throughout the entire body. (The Master Cleanse is a way of doing this.)

3) Ensuring the body gets adequate, good (non-tap) water (at least one ounce daily for every two pounds of body weight); non-iodized, unprocessed sea salt; and nutritional, raw vegetables (especially greens), fruits, sprouts, and soaked seeds and nuts to help the body rebuild the depleted nutritional reserves and organs.

4) Removing any stress-producing situations in the current environment.

5) Getting exercise and fresh air by lots of walking.

Now that you know these detox symptoms are only temporary and are milestones that you are becoming healthier, you will have the perspective to complete the cleanse and make it through. After you personally experience the gain you make after a detox day, you will actually begin to look forward to them, knowing that the next day will be a new plateau!

No detox symptoms

Many people wonder if they are eliminating toxins when they have no detox symptoms. The waste comes off in layers. So, you may not see anything happening for days and then have a detox day or see other results. I encourage you to continue through the full ten days. When I did my first cleanse (twenty days) I had nothing but bright yellow liquid for about a week in the middle of the twenty days. Then I had some semi-solid waste and felt great the next day. My wife discovered that just weighing yourself is not a good measure because she found that her body was changing shape and losing inches even when she was not losing weight.

**So, measure yourself before you start the cleanse, so you will have something to compare if your scale is not moving as fast as you want.

Severe detox symptoms

Have you taken a lot of medications? Are you overweight? Do you have allergies? All of these are indications of toxicity. More toxicity means you may have more detox symptoms the first few days relative to others who are in better condition. Sometimes a person is eating a good diet currently, but it is medications they took or an extremely bad diet long before their current cleanse that is causing the symptoms. The solution is to emphasize the elimination part of the Master Cleanse. Drink only six glasses of lemonade, ensure you are doing the laxative tea and salt water flush, drink at least half your weight in lemonade or water each day and take hot soaking baths of at least twenty minutes in two cups of Epsom Salt. If it gets really bad, discontinue the cleanse and use a slower method of detoxifying. (See the section "The Detox Diet Scale.") You can always do the cleanse again later. Remember, getting healthy is not a one-time event. It is a lifetime process.

"How About Only Five Days? Can We Make a Deal?"

Burroughs says to do the Master Cleanse for at least ten days at a time. Many people have asked if they could do it for less. My experience has shown that the days with the greatest chances for detox symptoms— remember, they are the milestones of progress—are the second, third, seventh and fourteenth (for those that go that long). The second and third days are fairly obvious. That is when the recent waste is being eliminated and thus is causing detox symptoms —cravings, irritability, etc. Notice that the seventh and fourteenth are seven days apart. At a talk given by Victoria Boutenko, a raw vegetarian speaker and writer, she showed a video of a live blood analysis that showed the clumping of red blood cells when people ate cooked food. She said it took seven days for the red blood cells to un-clump. Perhaps there is a seven-day cycle in the body that is triggered by the Master Cleanse. At any rate, I have noticed that the biggest benefits in mental clarity, serenity and focus come for most people after Day 8. The moral of the story? Stick with it for at least ten days, just like Burroughs says.

The Agitator and the Rinse Cycle

The Master Cleanse is designed to do two things: first to detoxify the body (remove toxins/poisons from the cells and organs in which they are embedded)—The Agitator—and then to eliminate those toxins from the body before they can be reabsorbed and poison the body once again—the Rinse Cycle. Just as a washing machine must incorporate both of those to be effective, so must any good cleanse.

Not eating any solid food permits your body to direct all of its digestive energy toward removing toxins from the cells and organs in which they are embedded. This process is aided by the six to twelve ten-ounce glasses of "lemonade" per day that you will drink on the Master Cleanse. The lemon juice helps to neutralize the acidic wastes and loosen them from where they are stored, and the cayenne pepper increases the blood flow to areas to be detoxified by dilating the blood vessels. The final part of the Agitator is the herbal laxative tea which stimulates the muscular contractions in the intestines, which "agitates" the contents and moves them toward final elimination.

Once the old toxic waste has been mobilized, you need the Rinse Cycle to eliminate it before it is reabsorbed. After the stomach has reduced the food you have eaten to a semi-liquid form, your body pushes it through the intestines where it absorbs what you have given it as nourishment. If the walls of the intestines are coated with years of waste, all daily nutrients must be absorbed through this coating and some of the old putrefied waste is carried into the blood stream.

Sadly, most "civilized" people tend to overeat, and to choose those things which are the most difficult to digest, such as meat and cheese. The final result of this kind of diet over decades is an accumulation of toxic waste, which is then re-absorbed into the blood. (You can read more about this in the excellent books by Dr. Norman W. Walker, such as *Colon Health: The Key to a Vibrant Life*, or *Become Younger*. Dr. Walker, by the way, lived to ninety-nine years of age, was mentally sharp and physically fit throughout his life, and is credited with the statement, "Death begins in the colon.")

The salt water flush is the Rinse Cycle and therefore vital. If you cannot drink the salt water flush in the morning, you should drink the laxative tea both evening and morning. (Take care not to drink more than two cups per day of pure senna tea or four cups per day of tea with 50 percent senna.) However, I believe that the agitator action of the laxative tea is different than the flushing action of the salt water flush and encourage people to do the salt water flush if at all possible. You would not wash your clothes in a washing machine with only an agitator and no rinse cycle, so why clean your digestive tract without a rinse cycle?

● The Master Cleanse Is Not for Everyone

The Master Cleanse is not for everyone. There are some people who should not even attempt it:

- People who are undergoing chemotherapy or have completed chemotherapy within the last six months must not do the Master Cleanse. Chemotherapy is based on the idea that administering a chemical poison will kill cancer cells before healthy cells. Under such treatment, a part of each dose accumulates in the body. (This information is from Max Gerson M.D., who developed a nutritional treatment for tuberculosis, cancer, and other degenerative diseases.) So, many treatments can accumulate a lethal dose if later released all at once. Therefore, such people must use a much slower detox method to avoid liver damage or worse.   (See "The Detox Diet Scale" below.)

- People who are recovering from major surgery or a severe wound— we are not talking a cut finger here—should not do the Master Cleanse. In order to build tissue, you must have extra protein. Since the Master Cleanse contains no protein, it will not support massive rebuilding of muscles. There is no danger from this lack of protein for a month or more, but such a lack will slow down healing. If you are recovering from major surgery, ask your surgeon when your healing is complete before doing the cleanse. People not in these categories—recovering from surgery or a severe wound—need not be concerned. People only lose one to two pounds of muscle mass no matter how long they do the cleanse because the body only burns muscle for energy for the first two days for women and three days for men.[3] Thereafter, it only burns fat and waste.

---

3   Fuhrman, Joel, M.D., *Fasting and Eating for Health*, St. Martin's Griffin, New York, NY, p. 12

This same process explains why athletes on the Master Cleanse do better with walking, jogging and swimming but not weight lifting and bodybuilding.

- Rapidly growing children should not do the Master Cleanse because they need protein for growth. The exception is if they are suffering from asthma or something similar. Several studies have shown fasting to be an effective treatment for such problems for people of all ages.[4]

- Opinion is divided on whether pregnant or nursing women should do the Master Cleanse. I have never heard of a single pregnant or nursing woman to be hurt by the cleanse, but in the spirit of "better safe than sorry," I began to say that pregnant or nursing women should not do the cleanse. Right after I published that in one of my newsletters, I got an email from a midwife who said she had thirty years of experience with the Master Cleanse being done by pregnant and nursing women and no one ever had a problem. Likewise, Stanley Burroughs and another Master Cleanse author, Tom Woloshyn, say that the Master Cleanse is fine for pregnant and nursing mothers. So, I will leave it up to you. (One clever woman who wanted to lose the extra weight she had gained while pregnancy and was going to be away from her baby for a cruise, stored enough of her breast milk for ten days and did the cleanse while her baby was taken care of by her mother using the stored breast milk.)

There are other people who may not be able to do all ten days of the cleanse. Someone who is much too toxic will find it nearly impossible not to eat. The body has a natural protective mechanism. They will go off the cleanse before the detoxification symptoms get to be too much. It is not dangerous for these people to do it, but they will benefit more from the slower methods of detoxification that create less detox symptoms. (See "Detox Diet Scale" below for a list.)

How do you know if you have a great deal of toxins? If you have two or more of the following, you may be too toxic:

- Allergic to "everything." Alternative medicine equates allergies with toxic reactions. If you are only allergic to bananas, that is probably

---

4 Papers submitted to the 2001 Fasting Therapy Conference, Ulan Ude, Russian Republic Of Buryatia, Ministry of Public Health Care

not too serious. If you are allergic to fifteen things, you need to take it easy.

- Very poor general health

- Multi-year history of strong medical or psychiatric drugs. Antibiotics every few years for infections are probably not much to worry about. Sleeping pills every night for ten years is another situation. If you are on or have had heavy psychiatric drugs, chemotherapy, etc. you should definitely check with your health professional.

- More than seventy pounds overweight. The body stores toxins in fat cells when it runs out of room in the liver. Serious overweight indicates there may be lots of toxins and waste to eliminate.

If you want to try the Master Cleanse even though you have such indicators, please follow the directions given in the section "If Detox Symptoms Become Unpleasant."

If you are taking blood thinners or high blood pressure medications, you should do the cleanse in coordination with your prescribing licensed health care practitioner. This is because the Master Cleanse will have similar effects as the medications, so if you are also taking medicine for these issues you may get a double whammy. So, be prepared to have your medication dosage reduced.

If Detox Symptoms Become Unpleasant

1. Drink only the minimum six drinks of lemonade each day.

2. Be sure to drink the herbal laxative tea every evening.

3. Drink enough additional water so that you have drunk at least one ounce of water or lemonade for each two pounds of body weight each day.

4. Be sure to do the salt water flush as given each morning.

5. Take a shower or long, soaking hot bath in two cups of Epsom Salt every day to draw out toxins.

The reasoning behind the recommendations above is to detoxify very lightly, but use the maximum amount of elimination methods so that whatever toxins are mobilized are quickly eliminated before being reabsorbed. Remember, you can do the Master Cleanse several times. So, do not push it.

Headaches

As I pointed out in "Detox Symptoms—The Good, the Bad and the Ugly," people who have heavy daily caffeine habits — coffee, tea, soda with caffeine, etc.— typically have bad headaches when they go cold turkey on the Master Cleanse. Realize it is the caffeine habit you are kicking and persevere. It does not make sense to go off the Master Cleanse in order to attempt to kick the habit without the enhanced elimination procedures. The longest I have known someone to have a headache was four days. Keep in mind if you have a headache for more than a day or so and never had a caffeine habit, this may signal other problems that you should not ignore. Therefore, you should quickly discover the cause.

When It Is Not All Coming Out as Planned

Not having any bowel movements? Here is a checklist to help you.

0. Some people expect they will have black rubbery eliminations on the Master Cleanse. Perhaps they have seen pictures of this on the Internet. This is produced by taking benonite clay and/or psyllium husks, which mechanically push the old wastes out rather than dissolve it. This is not what happens on the Master Cleanse. The lemonade and not eating will dissolve the old waste and toxins. As long as something is coming out, watery or not, do not worry.

1. Are you putting at least two level TEASPOONS of sea salt in the water each morning and having several urgent eliminations within an hour? If this is not happening, you have not got the right amount of salt in the water. For those on a heavy meat and/or cheese diet, it may take two or three days to work, but when you get the amount correct, the result is impossible to miss. You will have no doubt.

2. Are you mixing two tablespoons (one ounce) of fresh squeezed—not bottled—lemon juice into each drink or using these proportions for each batch and only mixing one day at a time?

3. Are you adding cayenne pepper to taste with each drink?

4. Are you drinking one cup of laxative tea each morning as well as each evening and the salt water flush to encourage more elimination? (Note: Discontinue the extra cup in the morning after you get things going.)

5. Are you eating or drinking anything else but lemonade, water, salt water, laxative herb tea and occasional mint tea?

6. Before this cleanse, did you have only one or two BMs per week? Being constipated before the Master Cleanse might mean a little longer before you see results.

7. Are you on any constipating medications? I am NOT suggesting you quit taking any prescribed medications. But they may delay the results of the Master Cleanse.

The Twelve Most Common Pitfalls

Having coached more than 2,000 people on the Master Cleanse and having more than 30,000 members of the Master Cleanse bulletin board that I ran for 10 years, I have seen 12 things trip people up over and over again while they were doing the Master Cleanse. These 12 are the most common. If you can avoid these, you will multiply your chances for success many times over.

1. Not getting all the correct written information before starting the cleanse

I know. You think I am saying this just because I want to sell my book. Well, I do want to sell my book. But that is not why I am saying this. Remember the children's game "telephone" where you whisper a message from one person to another? The message starts as "Say, Hi!" and ends as "I am at the post office."

The person who told you how to do it may or may not have remembered all the important information. They may not have the same concerns that you have. So they do not mention something important to you.

There are so many strange alterations. I cannot remember them all. But they have one thing in common. They will not get the great results that everyone else gets by following Stanley Burroughs' instructions. When you verbally tell your friend what you remember about the cleanse, you may be setting them up for a failure. And they may not remember exactly what you said either. I wish I had a dollar for everyone who says, "Oh! two teaspoons of sea salt in the salt water flush. I was trying to do it with two tablespoons!"

I have seen real people on the bulletin board talk about adding soy sauce to the salt water flush so it tastes like soup. (Soy sauce is protein and requires almost as much digestion as hamburger!) Another asked how many of the glasses of orange juice or vegetable soup are permitted each afternoon on the cleanse. (The answer? None!) Another woman talked about how she tried to handle her hunger with vegetable soup each afternoon! (That would start digestion going again and put her back on days two and three, the difficult ones over and over!)

To really help your friends, either give them the book or tell them to go buy it. They will value it more. And they will get the straight scoop. Their significant other might pick it up and help them or join them, too!

2. Not knowing what "detox" means

"Detox" is short for detoxify — meaning to eliminate toxins (poisons). It comes from "de-" meaning down or away, "toxin" meaning poison, and "-ify" meaning to make or do. So, "detoxify" means to make poisons come out or away (from the body). The toxins in our case are substances that your body can't absorb and use to rebuild the body. They actually harm your body's cells making you fat, tired, irritable, sick or, in extreme cases, dead.

So, when a person detoxifies, or detoxes, she or he is mobilizing the toxins stored in various places and eliminating them. When they are mobilized, the person may become tired, feel pain or aches, be irritable, develop rashes, etc. These symptoms (signs showing that something else exists) tell you that toxins have been mobilized. Next, they need to be eliminated. Once they are eliminated, you will feel better than before. The whole purpose of a cleanse is to eliminate toxins so that you feel better and are healthier than before.

3. Not knowing the detox symptoms

See "Detox Symptoms—the Good, the Bad and the Ugly."

4. Not knowing that detox symptoms will usually be gone or lessened with the next day's eliminations

Detox symptoms usually go away or at least lessen with the next day's eliminations. This is vital to understand because very few people can make it through ten straight days of cravings. But if you know those feelings will only last one more day, you can make it through all ten days of the Master Cleanse easily.

Too often, I hear of people quitting because they were discouraged and thought nothing was happening. First, their discouragement was a detox symptom — a sign something was happening. Second, they were only one morning away from feeling great and knowing they could do it. So, you can see how important it is to know about this pitfall.

The reverse of this is also important. If you are feeling sick and it doesn't go away or lessen after a few days, it is probably not a detox symptom. What then? If it's serious, consult your licensed health care practitioner. If it's not, either come off the cleanse and handle it or handle it as you think best.

5. Not doing all the elimination actions every day

If you really understand that detoxification is a two step process—mobilized, then eliminated—and that detox symptoms occur when these toxins are mobilized, but not yet eliminated, you will then understand the importance of doing all the elimination actions.

Sometimes a person can neglect one or another elimination action (salt water flush, laxative tea, drinking at least six lemonades a day) for a few days and feel no ill effects. Usually, that comes back to bite them later. Do all the elimination actions every day.

6. Not knowing the worst days are usually two, three and seven

I believe it is important to know which days are going to be the worst. For one thing, you will know that the entire Master Cleanse will not be that difficult. For another, you can look forward to better days. (By the way, people usually gain mental clarity and find that cooking for others does not bother them starting with day eight.)

It is amazing how many people quit on day two, three or seven! (Occasionally someone will be off by a day and have day one be the worst or day six.) In addition to not knowing which days are the worst, they usually do not know the detox symptoms and that they go away if the elimination actions are done each day.

I have observed that the body detoxes in seven-day cycles. When I did my 20-day cleanse, days two, three, seven and fourteen were the worst. I just recently finished a 28-day cleanse, but days 21 and 28 were fine. So, it is not always every seven days, but very frequently it is the case. I have found that each cleanse usually gets easier.

7. Confusing cravings with hunger

How do you tell the difference? If you really want a hamburger, but you would turn down a green salad, it is a craving. Why does it make any difference? When you realize you are feeling cravings, not hunger, you know they are just detox symptoms and will go away the next day.

8. Not drinking more lemonade or water when you feel hungry

Only one person in four reports any hunger on this cleanse. After checking to see if they are craving some food in particular, I tell them to drink more lemonade or water when they feel hungry. And their hunger usually disappears.

9. Eating or drinking anything else except lemonade, salt water, herbal laxative tea or mint tea while on the cleanse (except items prescribed by licensed health professionals)

A lady once posted to The Master Cleanse Bulletin Board that she kept feeling hungry. When I asked her to tell me exactly what she was doing, she told me she was drinking vegetable soup each afternoon! Of course, this was creating new cravings to torture her every day! So, rather than being done with cravings after the third day, she was continuing her cravings every single day of the cleanse!

Other people have asked about taking additional items, such as vitamins, supplements, chewing gum, sweetener for the tea, herbs, etc.

Hundreds of thousands of people have done The Master Cleanse since it was developed by Stanley Burroughs. It works. Just as written. The lemonade and maple syrup have all the necessary vitamins, minerals and calories to support the body for the duration of the cleanse.

10. Not using fresh-squeezed lemon juice

I am not saying you have to freshly squeeze the lemon (or lime) juice for each glass one at a time. If you have to go to work all day, you will have to make up enough for the whole day ahead of time. But try to make the last drink or two with freshly squeezed lemon juice after you get home. By the way, cayenne gets hotter the longer it sits. So, try to make two bottles for the day with three drinks in each bottle and put cayenne in the second bottle just before you are ready to drink it. (Cheap commercial plug: I sell two such bottles in an insulated bag for just this purpose in my web store at **www.TheMasterCleanse. com**/store.)

Do not use bottled, processed, or yesterday's juice. It is the enzymes (substances that encourage chemical changes) in the lemon juice that make it effective. These enzymes become less effective over time. By using freshly squeezed juice, your lemonade will be as effective as possible to help dissolve the old waste.

11. Going to social events during the first seven days

Something wonderful happens on day eight. Many people discover that cooking for others becomes much easier. A good friend, after day seven, helped a chef prepare grilled pork tenderloins for dinner and my friend on the cleanse was not bothered at all! (Usually, they gain mental clarity, too.)

However, before then, do not tempt yourself. Especially on days two, three and seven.

12. Being so focused on losing pounds that you do not notice you are losing inches

My wife discovered something interesting. She kept track of her measurements each day as well as her weight. A couple times her weight did not change. But she noticed that she was losing inches in places she wanted. Others talk about being able to fit into clothes they could not wear before even though they had not lost many pounds.

What to Expect Day by Day

These days may be off by one or two. For example, days two and three are usually the worst, but it could be days one and two.

Day 1:

Generally easy. One out of four people has trouble with the salt water flush. If so, you may substitute another cup of herbal laxative tea in the morning for the salt water flush. If you do, try the salt water flush after day seven as it gets easier after you eliminate some mucus. Most people find it much easier on their second or third Master Cleanse. People with caffeine habits may have headaches for the first few days. Four days is the longest I have heard for these headaches. Some people advise quitting caffeine before the cleanse to make it easier, but then you are doing it without the daily "agitator and rinse cycle" of the Master Cleanse which makes quitting easier and faster.

Days 2 and 3:

Usually the worst, although some people have no detox symptoms throughout the cleanse. It is important to remember during these two days that whatever you are feeling, it will lessen or go away with the next morning's eliminations. That is why I think Stanley Burroughs, the developer of the Master Cleanse, was such a genius. Fasting is a great way to rejuvenate the body. However, the toxins that are released can cause a person to feel quite bad. Burroughs added an "agitator and rinse cycle" (laxative tea and salt water flush) to remove toxins quickly so the detox symptoms stay manageable.

For the first two or three days, the body burns muscle for energy. On day three for women and day four for men, the body switches and begins to burn fat and waste for energy. Stick with it because when the body switches over, most people report it is well worth it—calmness, lack of tiredness, clear thinking, and a positive attitude, not to mention losing weight.

Days 4 to 6:

Most people report the benefits mentioned above. This is why I call the Master Cleanse the reset button for the body. Many people report their sense of smell is heightened.

Day 7:

A bit of a detox day, not as bad as days two and three, but possibly some detox symptoms of less intensity. At this point, the cleanse begins to eliminate older waste. These older toxins dissolve like layers of an onion.

Days 7 to 10:

Clear sailing like days four to six. Those who cook for their families generally find that by day eight it does not bother them to prepare food for others. They are beginning to have a sense of detachment from food. Other people find that they no longer are interested in watching TV or playing video games. Perhaps they enjoy soaking in the tub or reading. Many people report their body becoming more flexible, their skin becoming clearer, and less joint pain after this many days of the cleanse.

Day 14:

(if you go that far): Similar to day seven. Detox symptoms of less intensity than those on days two and three.

Day 16:

Some people experience a calm detachment toward food and life as well as a chance to reevaluate goals and plans. I discovered an intense desire to watch the Food Channel and smell other people's food, but I was not tempted to eat any of it—kind of like a Scratch 'n Sniff!

Days 21, 28, 35, etc.:

In my 17 or 18 Master Cleanses, I found detox days came every seven days or so. Sometimes I would be surprised by a solid elimination and would be amazed as I had not eaten anything for weeks!

The Detox Diet Scale

If you bring toxins out of storage faster than your body can neutralize and eliminate them, you will get a detox symptom or reaction. This is because the toxins can be reabsorbed before they are neutralized and eliminated.

The Master Cleanse is the second fastest method of detoxification. (A water-only fast is the fastest.) However, faster is not always better because it may be more than the body can handle. People with poor elimination or people with too many toxins need a slower method so their elimination system can keep up. In the case of those on or just off chemotherapy, this may possibly even cause harm.

I know a lady in New York who had a several-year history of strong medical drugs and was surprised that she was doing so well on the Master Cleanse until I discovered that she was using bottled, and thus pasteurized, lemon juice. (Pasteurization kills enzymes and severely reduces the effectiveness of the lemon juice.)

When she tried fresh-squeezed lemon juice, she had much stronger detox symptoms and had to switch to a slower method of detoxification. (By the way, this incident convinced me that bottled lemon juice is not acceptable for the Master Cleanse.)

Here is my scale of detoxifying actions ranked from fastest (1) to slowest (10). The fastest methods are good so long as you can tolerate the detox symptoms. If they are more than you can endure, see the section above "If Detox Symptoms Become Unpleasant" for actions you can take to reduce them for fast relief. If you still cannot handle them, switch to a slower method.

1. Pure-water fast (if done for more than a couple days, it is best done under a doctor's supervision)

2. The Master Cleanse, which permits working and aerobic exercise (as opposed to the pure-water fast, which sometimes requires bed rest.) Note: Bodybuilding exercise is not compatible with the Master Cleanse as there is no protein. You can live without protein for 40 days or longer, but you cannot build muscles without protein.

3. Fruit juice fast (fruits are detoxifiers)

4. Vegetable juice fast (veggies build up the body with vitamins, proteins and minerals)

5. Enemas or colonics (can be combined with all these other methods except the Master Cleanse)

6. 100 percent raw vegan diet

7. Predominantly raw vegan diet with the rest of the diet being cooked vegetarian food

8. 100 percent vegetarian diet without sugar or artificially preserved, colored, flavored, sweetened, or prepared foods

Drinking a quart of freshly made green smoothie every day (Go to the "Raw Food Recipes" page on my website **www.TheMasterCleanse. com** for the recipe.)

9. Drinking a pint of freshly made green smoothie every day

10. Soaking in a hot Epsom Salt bath (two cups to a regular sized tub) at least three times a week for twenty minutes, which can also be combined with any of the above

Part IV

Your Master Cleanse Journal

Date Started: _____ Weight: _____

Measurements: Chest: _____ Waist: _____ Hips: _____ Thighs: _____

Energy level on a scale of one to ten (one being the lowest): _____

	Optional: 1 cup of herb laxative tea in a.m.	32 oz. water with 2 tsps non-iodized sea salt	No. of 10-ounce lemonade drinks (6 – 12)	Evening 1 cup of herb laxative tea	Comments (wins or detox symptoms)
Night before	N/A	N/A	N/A		
Day 1					
Day 2					
Day 3					
Day 4					
Day 5					
Day 6					
Day 7					
Day 8					
Day 9					
Day 10					

Date Finished: _____ Weight: _____

Measurements: Chest: _____ Waist: _____ Hips: _____ Thighs: _____

Energy level on a scale of one to ten (one being the lowest): _____

Part V

The Master Cleanse
Discussion Bulletin Board

For those not familiar with the idea of an Internet bulletin board (also called a forum), it is a discussion group organized much like a public bulletin board where anyone is free to post their comments for all to see and others are free to post responses to those already posted or to start another topic. Because it is on the Internet, you can see the responses as soon as someone posts them. This allows people to give immediate feedback, to answer questions and to give support for one another.

In this last section, I have reprinted various questions and comments from my Master Cleanse bulletin board, which operated for 10 years from 2004 to 2014; the majority came from 2004. I have altered the names of the people writing these comments to provide privacy. I have kept them consistent, so you can see who said what and compiled these comments within the topics to which they apply. The topics have been alphabetized for your convenience.

As far as content, I have had to take some editorial license to edit the topics and postings within them. This is for the most part because of sheer volume. If I had not, this book would be nearly twice as long without adding any new ideas. I have tried to give you an idea of what what that bulletin board was like, with its feeling of community and support. Unfortunately by 2014, huge volumes of automated spam made it difficult to maintain the value of the board and its sense of community. Even the professionals I hired were unable to prevent or automatically eliminate the spam and I was forced to close the bulletin board permanently.

Acid/alkaline balance/pH?

Peter
Much attention has been focused lately on alkalizing the body. The need for this can be clearly seen when you realize that meat, sugar, flour, and cooked foods produce acid in the body when digested. Raw fruits,

vegetables, seeds and some nuts produce an alkaline condition. This includes lemons, which are acid before they are eaten, but produce an alkaline result when eaten. When you fast, the body begins to mobilize and eliminate the acidic toxins. Therefore the urine pH during a fast becomes acidic. Calcium, magnesium, potassium and sodium (alkaline minerals) are used by the liver to neutralize the acidic toxins before they are eliminated. This is the reason you have to have alkaline mineral reserves to do the Master Cleanse. After the cleanse, the body is in more of an alkaline state.

After the Cleanse

Peter
After you are done with the cleanse, your body naturally will be inclined to eat more raw fruits and vegetables. So, be sure to check out the recipes page at **www.TheMasterCleanse.com**.

Person No. 1
I am amazed at how my body/mind only wants to consume raw fruits and veggies. Although I have gained three of the fourteen pounds back, I still am one pant size smaller than I was before starting the MC. This statement may be a little far fetched to say but I believe that once the body has gotten rid of toxins, it instinctively craves the fresh, live foods that it so desperately needs to sustain itself and to heal itself. After all, humans have the teeth of herbivores not carnivores.

Person No. 2
I'm on Day 10. Had my one orange for ten minutes, just sat and chewed. Felt very good. I am going to try juicing for another week, then go to raw food. Thanks for all the support and information along the way. A person can't do these things without others. May God bless all of you for your help.

Person No. 3
I am on Day 12 and felt it would emotionally serve me to stop at this point. My tongue was covered with white fuzzy stuff and then when I brushed my teeth, it was completely pink.

I have been reading that after the cleanse I will want to eat fruits and veggies. However, I feel inclined to go towards my old favorites, meat and dairy. Is that a sign that something is wrong or I did it wrong? Also, I was wondering what you know about salt flushing once or twice a week after the cleanse.

Peter

If you did the cleanse and you felt better, you didn't do it wrong. First, take probiotics when you resume eating solid food. Follow the directions on the label. It will help prevent cravings. Then if you want meat or dairy, go ahead, but try to include a salad meal each day as well. You can always do another cleanse.

A fellow I met told me he had done the cleanse three times. After the first, he was no longer interested in red meat. After the second cleanse, he found he liked raw vegetables more. After the third, he was no longer interested in meat and wanted organic vegetables. That covered three years of his life.

The salt water flush may be done after the MC whenever you feel it will help. Be sure to do it on an empty stomach, though. The MC lemonade is recommended as a daily breakfast drink. My wife and I use salt water flushing whenever we feel we need to wash out our digestive tract after an occasional dinner out with friends. It works great. A healthy diet is a lifelong process, not a one time event.

Person No. 3

Thanks for the quick response. The cleanse was great and I feel so much better. I was wondering what juicing meant. I have read that a few people juice for a week or so after the cleanse. Is that orange juice, grapefruit, or lemonade?

Also, I have found that I love the way I look and feel. How can I prevent my weight coming back? I lost eighteen pounds. I know that diet and food play an important part but is there anything else? This bulletin board has been a life saver. Thanks so much!!!

Peter

Juicing can include a pure juice fast, drinking occasional vegetable juices to rebuild the body, drinking occasional fruit juices to cleanse the body, and everything in between. When I finish a cleanse, I find I want vegetable and fruit juices along with other fresh, raw vegetables, fruit, nuts, and seeds. Others may want nothing but juices for a few days. It's all a matter of what your body wants.

To prevent weight coming back, be sure you eat at least 50 percent fresh raw vegetables and fruit and if you do eat meat or dairy, do a salt water flush occasionally. In addition, I recommend doing the Master Cleanse at least twice a year. Weight gain is all about what you eat. If you eat foods that your body sees as toxins, the body will protect itself by making mucus to line the digestive tract and store the toxins in the body fat. That is just how it is. Eat junk and get fat. If you eat real food, nutritious food, you will lose to an ideal weight and not gain it back at all. There you go: Total control of your weight and health!

Person No. 67
I appreciate all your time and input. I am now off the cleanse and started with orange juice and have moved into veggies. I am going slow so I can incorporate more fruit and veggies in my diet. However, I am experiencing gas. Is this common and what can I do about it?

Peter
I haven't run into that after the cleanse. I did experience gas the first time I did the cleanse around Day 4. I thought it was gas from the old waste being dissolved by the lemonade. It went away after a couple days.

Burroughs says if you have gas you should continue the cleanse for "several more days."

Agave Nectar vs. Maple Syrup
I had a phone call from a lady who told me she had done a Master Cleanse with agave and didn't feel like it had done as much as maple syrup and wanted to do the MC again with maple syrup. When I researched it, I discovered that agave has to be heated to approximately 140 degrees to cause it to become sweet. (It is not sweet naturally.) That causes it to be about 85 percent fructose, which makes it higher in fructose (42–55 percent) than high fructose corn syrup (HFCS). A 2007 study showed a link between HFCS, obesity and liver problems.[1] Maple syrup is about one-half percent fructose according to the USDA National Nutrient Database. In addition, agave contains about a third of the potassium in a similar amount of maple syrup. I also know that Tom Woloshyn, who also wrote a book about the Master Cleanse, discourages people from using agave for the Master Cleanse and cites another practitioner who discourages people from using agave for more than ten days because it led to demineralization.

---

1 Paper presented by Brent Tetri, M.D., professor of internal medicine at Saint Louis University Liver Center at the Digestive Diseases Week conference, 2007

Anti-depressants

Person No. 4
After getting everyone else started on this, I am finally ready to do it. I had to wean myself off anti-depressant medication first. It took two weeks.

Peter
Congratulations on getting yourself off the anti-depressant.

For those who want to go off anti-depressants and don't have medical/professional assistance, I recommend going to www.TheRoadBack.org. They have a free book on how to come off anti-depressants safely and a list of doctors for those who need more help. I do not recommend doing the cleanse while on a strong anti-depressant. They are very toxic and can create severe detox symptoms during the cleanse.

Bentonite, Psyllium, Herbs, Colon Cleansers During the Cleanse

Person No. 6
Hi, all. I recently read about doing several Bentonite and Psyllium Husk shakes per day with a cleanse. Supposedly it helps with bowel movements and removing mucus layers in the intestine. Has anyone else heard of this or used this method along with the Master Cleanse? All responses are welcome! Thanks a bunch.

Person No. 7
I've never tried them during this particular cleanse but I have used them with other cleanses (juicing and such) and had good results. After I finished this cleanse (two days ago) and started eating whole foods again I introduced psyllium and organic ground flax seeds in my diet to help my colon get back into shape. If you're going to do this, drink plenty of water before and afterward since it absorbs lots of it once it's down. Personally, I find that using the senna tea for a long period of time is like trying to run five miles after not wearing your shoes for a few months.

It's probably best to stick to the program to get the best results. However, I would like to hear from others who have done this during the cleanse and hear their results.

Person No. 8
From what I have read, it is not good to stay on senna tea for long term because it irritates your colon. That is why it works for the cleanse. Psyllium husk is not good to be on because it robs your colon of water and the most important thing you need for good bowel movements is at least eight glasses a day. I am reading a book right now called *Your Body's Many Cries for Water*. The author (F. Batmanghelidj, M.D.) states that all diseases can be cured if the body has sufficient water. A lot of the stuff he says makes sense. So even though I go to the bathroom a lot anyway, I am trying to drink eight glasses of water a day.

Person No. 9
In doing research about the Master Cleanse, I found a website that talks about "The Ultimate Fast." It sounds like the Master Cleanse except that certain products are added: one for parasites, something called a Colon Cleanse tablet, and psyllium and bentonite products. It has links to buy the products, too. It goes for eight days and then with modifications for ninety days.

I was just wondering if anyone knew if these steps were really necessary for complete and thorough cleansing, including the elimination of parasites. I thought psyllium was a form of fiber, although I could be wrong, but if I'm not, that means your colon really wouldn't be "resting" throughout the cleanse, right? I am interested in the bentonite thing, because the website I found claims it's the only thing known to remove plaque from the walls of the intestines and colon. Having Crohn's disease, I think that would be especially beneficial.

I'm doing my shopping for the cleanse tomorrow and wasn't sure if I needed this added stuff. I'm excited! Thank you again.

Person No. 8
Sounds to me like they are trying to sell you their products that you don't need. Just follow the Master Cleanse as written and it will get rid of the toxins and gunk in your body.

Person No. 9
That's what I figured, too. I'm still going to research that bentonite stuff, though. I'm curious now! Thanks.

Person No. 8
Yeah, the bentonite sounds interesting since they say that is the only thing that will remove the plaque from the walls of the intestines. I checked the site more thoroughly and they also promote the Awareness

products which I used when I started the Hallelujah Diet. They are very expensive and really not necessary. You can do more with the Master Cleanse and eating raw fruits, vegetables, nuts and seeds when you are done. However, I wonder if the bentonite will clean more of the mucus buildup so someone doesn't need to do a twenty-day cleanse to really get rid of stuff. My husband just did twenty days (I only made it six) and he probably wouldn't go twenty days again.

Peter

After I did my first twenty-day cleanse a year ago, I decided to do the Schultz herbal cleanse with herbs, psyllium and bentonite clay. I did it for ten days and didn't think it did anything for me as I was already quite clean from the Master Cleanse.

As to whether psyllium, bentonite clay, herbs or colon cleansers are the only way to remove old waste on the colon walls, I go by the appearance of the tongue. Chinese doctors have used the tongue to diagnose internal organs for thousands of years and I am amazed at what it reveals during the cleanse! When I checked tongue color, I discovered that the two people I know who have eaten a pure raw veggie, fruit, nut and seed diet have perfectly pink tongues. I have also produced a perfectly pink tongue after adding an ounce of wheatgrass juice to my raw food diet for seven days right after a seventeen-day cleanse. Based on that, I would say that colon cleanses, psyllium, etc. are not the only way to remove old waste on your colon walls. Not only does the MC cleanse the colon, it also gives the colon and digestive system a rest to rejuvenate.

Adding anything to the Master Cleanse weakens it because fasting is what gives it power. Fasting has been used for thousands of years to rejuvenate the body and focus the mind. Jesus, Moses, Ghandi, Buddha, Mohammed, Socrates, Plato, and Hippocrates (The Father of Western Medicine) all fasted and recommended fasting. Allan Cott, M.D., wrote *Fasting: The Ultimate Diet*, a million-copy bestseller, in 1975 on the benefits of fasting. So, adding anything reduces its effectiveness. Stick to the program as developed by Stanley Burroughs to get the best results. This does NOT mean discontinue any PRESCRIBED medications.

Beyond 10 Days

Person No. 10

I am on Day 8 and feel great. My joints are all moving freely and my arthritic pains are just about gone. I was prepared to stay on the cleanse for as long as it took for my tongue to turn pink, but it is pink already.

So, I will probably just stay for the ten days unless there is a further benefit I don't know about. Thanks for all your assistance, Peter.

Peter

I would divide the benefits of going beyond the tenth day into two categories. The first are spiritual in nature. Although temporary, I found a sense of serenity, an increased ability to face and handle problems, the ability to face stress without handling it with food, seeing your life goals in perspective and the absence of a desire to eat "bad" food even while I could appreciate and enjoy the smell of it. The idea of consuming something that would be bad for my body even though it smelled good was like the idea of eating a scratch n' sniff sticker. You would not even think of it.*

The second category of gain is physical improvement. I will tell you that people I know who have done more than twenty days, say the benefits came from the additional days

For the record, I occasionally eat unhealthy things just for the fun of it. However, the vast majority (more than 90 percent) of food I eat is fresh, raw real food with nutritional value and no added preservatives, additives, colors, poisons, etc. I have also leaned that when I do eat "bad" food I can just do the salt water flush the next day, if I feel bad. I also know I can hit the body's "reset button" by doing a Master Cleanse, which for me and others I know, gets the body back to wanting healthy food and juices.

Boredom

Person No. 6

One acute symptom I am feeling during this fast is boredom now that I taken myself off eating, I'm experiencing a peaceful sort of tiredness where I don't feel like doing much of anything. This is Day 1 of my cleanse. I figure this must be one of those uncomfortable times in life where you feel alone, when in truth you really are not. So, besides reading and watching TV, what are people doing when they're bored and really want to eat something solid? How do you keep your mind preoccupied with anything other than food? Any input would be greatly appreciated. Thanks!

Person No. 11

I went to Google and typed in "I am bored" and hit the search button! Ok, that was when I was desperate! Aside from that, I read. It makes time fly. Or I paint, or I practice my bass, or I go take a little catnap.

Mainly I have been Googling "Master Cleanse" to find out as much as I can about people's experience on this fast. Oh, and I can't forget, I spend a lot of time trying to get my friends to do this with me! Then we can all whine to each other and I wouldn't feel so alone. Finding this site helped a lot though. I think I will probably do some Pilates today. Not for boredom but to give my body some much needed exercise! Good luck with the cleanse, stick with it! I'm on Day 4 and I am already feeling great! I can only imagine Day 10!

Person No. 6

Thanks for responding to this topic! I thought maybe I was the only one losing my mind over this thing! This is Day 2 for me and I can honestly say that I feel good. The bored-out-of-my-skull, listless feelings I had yesterday, are not present right now. I don't feel lethargic. I can move again! And my mind isn't totally on food today! So Day 2 is definitely better for me than Day 1. Oh, by the way, as far as being bored is concerned, I think I also drove Google crazy typing in any word in relation to the Master Cleanse that I thought might help me along, i.e. "Master Cleanse journey," "Master Cleanse journal," etc. To combat boredom I started a journal, wrote a ton of poetry, laughed out loud at mindless sitcoms, fell asleep on a really good novel a couple of times, and, of course, prayer and more prayer.

Person No. 11

That's wonderful! It's great that you are keeping an upbeat attitude! Just think of all the good this is doing to your body! Last night I had a very emotional AND spiritual detox experience. I pray every night before bed of course, but last night was different. I was emotionally overcome and I cried and cried, not because I was sad. I think it was because so much clutter is being removed from my body and my mind. It's hard to explain accurately but suffice it to say, that I felt like a weight had been lifted off my shoulders when I was done. I dedicated my ten-day fast to God, so it makes it a little easier to resist the temptation to give in. I just think of all He has given me— ten days is nothing in comparison! Anyway, best of luck to you on this cleanse! Update me on any other ways you are combating boredom!

Peter

It sounds like you two are doing great on the cleanse. Boredom is one of the detox symptoms. When you get past the first two or three days, you will feel wonderful. That is your natural state. Boredom is the result of toxins in your body.

Person No. 12

What great wonderful things I just read in this topic! I just want to say that I had a dream I kicked a soccer ball in the goal. This may not sound important to you, but as a child of elementary age I played soccer and was not ever really good. I am glad I played soccer because I believe sports are wonderful for young children and I think being good at sports has to do with practice as well as being in a confident mindset.

Anyway I kept having these recurring dreams that disturbed me for many years of adulthood. The dreams were of me playing soccer as a child and never getting the ball in the goal. I would miss the ball or mess up, feeling frustrated when I woke up.

So, this dream of succeeding at getting the ball in the goal was an accomplishment I've desired. Though I may never be a great soccer player physically, the dream was enough to satisfy my subconscious mind.

Thank you for your postings. I feel great and look forward to a detox of my body—and mind as well!

Bowel Movements

Person No. 13

Is everyone here using organic lemons? I had some conventional lemons left from before I started my fast, which never seemed to give me problems. So, that is what I have been using. But I am starting to think this is part of what is making this cleanse so painful for me. My butt is on fire when I eliminate now. I'm wondering if the chemicals in the conventional lemons are just too harsh on an empty stomach like this. Tomorrow I will get some organics.

Peter

The burning poops are caused by the toxins leaving your body. Toxins are acid. They burn. The first cleanse I did was so bad I had to put some vitamin E on my butt for Days 2–5. By then, the burning stopped and only came back on the seventh day.

Person No. 13

Thanks for your reply. I guess I'll just have to deal with the burning, but I am going to switch to organic lemons anyway. No point in putting more chemicals back in my body while I'm trying to get them out to begin with.

Person No. 1

Now that you mention hot poop—before I completed the ten-day MC, I did a thirty-six-hour MC because I had never fasted before. Afterwards, I felt really great and ate raw fruit and veggies and fresh juice for five days. Then I started the ten-day MC. It was the evening of Day 1 of the ten-day MC that I had a really hot BM. I thought I was literally eliminating hot flames from my butt. It was much hotter than a burning sensation. Then I did some research and found out that my body was probably eliminating acid toxins. WOW!

Person No. 14

Just wanted to clarify something. I usually have a BM on awakening which I presume is from the laxative tea. I then drink the SWF (salt water flush) and within an hour I have as many as five BMs. Should I be having more BMs throughout the day? I am not, but reading other people's experiences, they seem to have far more eliminations. Am I doing it right? I would be grateful for any thoughts on this and experiences that anyone else is having. Thanks a lot.

Person No. 15

I'm having the exact same problem, only worse. I'm on my third day and am not having any BMs throughout the day. I haven't from the beginning. I'm only having the runny yellow liquid in the morning—pretty gross. Plus, the laxative tea is giving me severe cramps in the middle of the night. The back of the package says you should stop taking it if you find there's discomfort, so I don't know what to do. I'm following the directions exactly. What I want to know is, will this change? I don't think I should go for ten days if this persists.

Peter

Here is my experience with four Master Cleanses over a one-year period. For the first few days of the first cleanse, I had only one semi-solid BM in the morning. After a few days, I'd have one very watery BM first thing in the morning and then several (four or so) watery flushes from the salt water starting thirty to sixty minutes after drinking it and lasting for an hour or two. I had no more BMs after that for the rest of the day. After Day 10 on the first fast (it was a twenty-day fast), I might have had one or two more small, very watery BMs during the rest of the day.

On later cleanses, I would have more watery flushes after only two or three days, but none after that during the day. The watery ones are always bright yellow. Usually there are small brown mucousy flakes that I believe are the broken down remains of older waste.

Liquid BMs are the usual on the cleanse. Solid ones are unusual after the first day, although you could have semi-solid ones on later days because the intestines detox in layers. Therefore you will have periods of runny BMs and possibly semi-solid ones later. The waste of a lifetime comes off in layers and takes quite a while to dissolve if you have been eating a diet heavy in meat and dairy. But don't worry, the cayenne and lemon juice WILL dissolve it.

**Concerning abdominal cramps from the laxative tea, when you get past Day 5 or so, due to less waste in the intestines, you can feel the intestinal contractions. At times, they are uncomfortable.

They can be handled by:

1) Using an herbal tea that is a combination rather than pure senna tea;

2) Drinking water or lemonade to give the intestines something to push along rather than just cramp up the muscles; and

3) Reducing the amount of tea to half a cup and then filling it with water so that it is diluted by half.

These contractions are occasional for me and when they are present they are uncomfortable, but not painful, except for one or two days when they were painful for perhaps fifteen minutes before I went to the bathroom. Then the cramps disappeared completely.

If yours are truly painful and last more than two days and the above three things don't handle, then you should probably discontinue the herbal laxative tea. However, then you MUST be doing the salt water as I do NOT recommend anyone do this cleanse without elimination aids. There are just too many toxins released.

Person No. 14
Peter, thanks for such reassuring information. Instinctively I felt what I was experiencing was right but when you start reading other people's posts, the doubts creep in. Your experiences with the cleanse pretty much mirror my own. I now feel okay. I'm just starting Day 5. I have only had minimal weight loss but my body feels a lot different. (I was near to my ideal weight any way.) I woke up at 6:30 (with a little bit of help from two small kids) and didn't feel at all groggy. Wow, that is a new experience for me. Overall I am feeling just great. I'm not finding the Master Cleanse a picnic by any means (I'm really craving fruit and veggies) but it is so doable and I am loving the results. Thanks so much to all for your advice and encouragement.

Person No. 15

Sounds like you are doing great on the MC, too. I guess logically there wouldn't be much bowel activity through the day as you eliminate most of it with the flush. Also, I guess the word "flush" suggests something fast and complete. I suppose reading other people's comments can be good if it backs up what you are experiencing, but it can cast doubts when it doesn't. I think you and I are doing just great and probably having textbook reactions. Perhaps, we both need to have more faith in our bodies to do the right thing. I know I do. Good luck with the rest of the cleanse.

Person No. 12

Ok, I've been reading and reading all these comments, questions and responses. I am a little confused on the bowel movements. I am on Day 4 today and my bowel movement (diarrhea-like liquid) is early in the morning. After that, I drink the salt water and then my movement is completely water, the color of lemonade.

In some responses, it says the solid bowel movements may come around Day 8-10 according to the person's body and toxins. However, in others it says if you continue to have diarrhea after Day 4 or 5, you should seek a doctor and stop the cleanse.

I have not had a solid movement since I started this cleanse! I went on this diet after coming off the Atkins diet for about a week or so. So, I think I am really stopped up with cheese and meat!

Also my diet has been bad for a long time and I worked in a bar for many years and drank alcohol regularly and smoked when I drank. I know I have lots of toxins to be released. Is the one-time morning movement of diarrhea-like liquid followed by the water release normal?? I know the tea is causing my early diarrhea-like bowel movement and the salt water is causing the flush, but is there hope for a solid movement? How long should I wait?

Person No. 13

I can't speak from experience much, since this is my first time doing the cleanse, but if you are just coming off Atkins you are VERY stopped up. I did Atkins a couple of years ago and I was constantly constipated. I am probably still getting rid of stuff from back then, or will be during this cleanse.

I'm sure the moderator will reply, and you should listen to what he says above all, because he's done this cleanse many times. But I would say, if you feel okay, keep it up till you get a solid movement. That one movement of diarrhea per day is probably not enough to harm you as long as you are drinking enough fluids to replace what you lose—and on this cleanse you should be. I think you will eventually see results. It's just going to take some time for that impacted stuff to break apart and come out.

Person No. 12
Thanks. I appreciate the response. I was beginning to get worried. I have been a little constipated from Atkins so I will wait it out. Other than that, I feel fine. I am cold a lot with chills and a little stuffy. That's about it. My energy has not really increased much, but my mornings are definitely NOT groggy! I am sooo looking forward to the brighter days ahead. I have had some very strange dreams—dreams that I am conquering a fear I had since I was kid!! I think that is a definite enlightenment from this diet! I hope you are doing well too. I have read your postings. Good luck.

Person No. 1
Hang in there. Day 2 through 4, I had flu-like symptoms. I had liquid, mucousy movements as you described. Then on Day 6, I eliminated some intestinal-shaped matter about three to four feet long. No more really extensive toilet inspections for me after that! It was pretty scary. Then, I had a few more days of liquid, mucousy movements. Later on Days 8, 9 and 10, I eliminated stuff that smelled like the real thing. (So, I guess it was the real thing.) After that, I extended my cleanse beyond the minimum ten-day recommendation.

I have read that the intestines detox in layers. So your intestines will remove any old, built-up layers over time. Therefore you will have periods of liquid and mucousy BMs and then mucousy and solid BMs. Based on my experience this is true. Therefore it is very important to drink the correct lemonade formula, use the salt water cleanse in the mornings and laxative tea at night before bed and drink additional water during the day as well.

Every person's body is not the same. Hang in there and do not quit! Your body is just detoxing.

Good luck to you all! I'll be back the last week in March.

Person No. 12
Thanks to you all. Cool deal! I feel better now. Can't wait to pass the mass!

Person No. 11
I am on Day 9 and I have yet to have any solid BMs. Mine are all runny. However, they're not only liquid. There is stuff in there that needed to get out. I am wondering if I will have any solid BMs at all! If I don't, is that bad? Also, it is not recommended to drink senna tea for more than seven days. Any suggestions? I just can't keep the salt water down, even with warm water.

Peter
Re: Runny vs. solid BMs. All the others have been quite correct in their postings. The waste of a lifetime comes off in layers and takes quite a while to dissolve if you've been eating a diet heavy in meat and dairy. But don't worry, the lemonade WILL dissolve it.

[There is more about senna tea in the "Laxative tea" topic below.]

Person No. 12
Thank you, Peter, for your time, energy and advice. You are making a world of a difference in my life and many others! We all appreciate it.

Person No. 13
When I eliminate, the liquid that comes out has consistently been a neon yellow color so far. Is this acid or bile and are other people having this happen? (I know acid is coming out. I wasn't sure if that is what contributed to the color though.)

Peter
To my knowledge, it always happens. I believe the yellow is from bile.

Person No. 16
It's from the vitamin Bs in the maple syrup. Vitamin B6 and sometimes B12 causes your pee to be highlighter yellow.

Person No. 13
Ah, danke (thank you).

Person No. 17
It is true that B vitamins cause your pee to be yellow, but I think we are referring to the yellow color of our BM liquid. I tend to agree with Peter that it is the bile or perhaps the lemonade?

Peter
Probably bile, rather than lemonade. There's just not enough yellow color in the lemons.

It is true that B12 and other B vitamins turn your pee yellow, but I've never seen them turn my BMs yellow.

Person No. 12
My BMs have gotten darker and darker as the days have gone by. I am happy with that. They have a little more texture, but still liquid. Gosh, I haven't had one thing solid to eat in ten days and it's still flowing out. Amazing! How funny to chat about our private pooping experiences. I love it!

Person No. 18
I'm on Day 7 and I'm still amazed too. Mine also gets darker and darker each day. I guess the deeper the "do," the darker the hue. Okay, that's the lemonade talking. Not only is it funny to be talking about our bowel movements, but I think I've become borderline obsessive about them. Can't read enough of this stuff.

Person No. 13
Yeah, I'm obsessive too. My favorite part is looking in the toilet to see what came out each time. It makes the pain I go through (that tea makes me hurt) worth it. Boy, I am not pleased to know what was in me all that time, but I am so pleased to see it come out.

Mine is not getting darker and darker like that, though. It was really dark the first couple days. Now I am just getting these little bits and pieces of things (mostly old rotten meat—yuck!). Maybe I got the big initial stuff out and now I am just chipping away at the rest. That is what I hope. Today is Day 8. I haven't had a big mass come out since Day 2.

Bowel Movements Not Happening

Person No. 19
Hi. Today is my third day on the cleanse, and I haven't had a BM since Day 1. Because I didn't go yesterday, I increased my salt to three teaspoons today, but it still didn't work. Any suggestions? Thanks.

Peter
Some people come to the Master Cleanse from the Atkins diet and have eaten heavily of dairy and meat and white flour products. Worse, they

may have been taking medicines and many of them are constipated as a side effect. Sometimes it takes a few days.

Just ensure you are doing the laxative tea at night and the salt water flush in the morning and six to twelve drinks of lemonade with fresh lemon juice as instructed in the book. Then if you still are not eliminating, add a single cup of laxative tea first thing in the morning as well. Beyond that, don't worry. The cleanse will work it out, believe me.

Person No. 16
I'm in the beginning of Day 3 and I've only made one bowel movement on Day 1. This morning I drank half a quart of the salt water flush. I couldn't muster it all. I did the herbal tea last night. Why isn't there any elimination?

Peter
Some people may be taking medicines and many of them make a person constipated as a side effect. Sometimes it takes a few days.

1. People who eat SAD (the Standard American Diet of 100 percent meat, dairy, cooked food, no raw vegetables, and very few raw fruits) get "plugged up" and it can take two or three days before the full quart salt water flush begins to eliminate.

2. Not drinking at least six ten-ounce drinks of lemonade a day (or more for larger people) makes for less eliminations.

3. The salt water flush not only produces several liquid eliminations starting within thirty to sixty minutes, but also provides the colon with liquid to promote later eliminations and make them easier.

So, be patient, ensure you are doing the laxative tea at night and the salt water flush in the morning, and drink six to twelve lemonades with fresh lemon juice as instructed. Then if you still are not eliminating, add a single cup of laxative tea first thing in the morning as well. Beyond that, don't worry. The cleanse will work it out, believe me.

By the way, some people think if they eliminate only a bright yellow liquid that it doesn't count as a bowel movement. I consider anything that comes out the "back end" as a bowel movement.

Person No. 20
Hi. This is the first time I have tried the MC. I am in Day 3 and I am having a bit of a problem. I am not hungry or anything but I am not having any BMs. Yesterday I had a small one but that's it. I am not

taking the salt water because it makes me vomit, but I am drinking the laxative tea. What can I do?

Person No. 21

I'm a newbie too, but I'm on Day 10. I've read that if you can't tolerate the salt water flush that you can do the laxative tea morning and night. Also you need to be sure you're drinking enough water in addition to the lemonade. I usually alternate water with the lemonade. That should help move things along. When you tried the salt water flush did you use pure sea salt with no additives? It is much easier to tolerate than regular salt. I had been using sea salt, but I noticed after reading more closely that it had non-clumping agents. I bought some without that and it is much easier to drink. I drink it with a straw really quickly so I don't have to really taste it. The first time I did it I nearly threw up, but now I'm used to it, especially since I've been using the straw.

Person No. 20

Thanks. I think that the problem is that I am not drinking enough water. I did use sea salt—the only kind that was available to me from a health food store. I am going to try to drink more water.

Person No. 3

I am on Day 4 and still have a sinus infection. I am starting to have some BMs but not much. I am going back to my herbal colon cleanse. The tea did nothing for me. I really am tired. My spirits are high and I feel pretty good all around. However, I know that my real detox hasn't started yet.

Peter

I'm sorry to hear that you needed to go back to your herbal colon cleanse. For the sake of my education on the cleanse, can you answer a few questions to help me know exactly where it went wrong for you?

Can you tell me exactly how you had been mixing your lemonade?

How much of it you were drinking per day?

How you mixed your salt water?

Did you do it (salt water flush) every day?

What herbal laxative tea you used?

Did you drink it every night?

Did you take or eat anything else while on the cleanse?

What was your diet like before the cleanse?

Do you take any medications? (You don't need to be specific as to which ones.)

How long have you been taking the herbal colon cleanse?

Person No. 3 never answered these questions. but they are quite effective in locating why people are having trouble. In my experience, such trouble usually is for one of two reasons. They are not following the instructions, possibly from misunderstanding them, or they are actually doing fine, but had different ideas of what should happen.

You can check if you are not following instructions by answering the questions above and then comparing them to the written instructions to see if you misunderstood the instructions. Likewise, you can check your ideas of what should happen by reading these questions and answers.

Breaking the Fast—Very Important

Peter
The longer you are on the MC, the more important it is to break it correctly. People who have only been on it for two or three days generally have no problem breaking it, provided they drink orange juice for the first day after they stop drinking lemonade. After ten days, you should follow the procedure for breaking the cleanse because going straight back to food can make you nauseous and/or cause stomach pain. After seventeen days, correctly breaking the Master Cleanse is important and after thirty or more days it is VERY important. I did it wrong once and had nausea and stomach pains for more than an hour. Here are the Instructions for breaking it:

For vegetarians: Slowly drink as many glasses of orange juice as you want for each of the first two days. You may dilute the juice if you like or if you have any digestive problems. On the third day, drink orange juice in the morning, eat fresh fruit for lunch and have a fruit or raw vegetable salad for dinner.

For non-vegetarians: Slowly drink several glasses of orange juice for the first day and through the afternoon of the second. You may dilute the juice if you like or if you have any digestive problems. For dinner on the second day, drink mostly the broth of a vegetable soup you make yourself that afternoon from several different vegetables, such as carrots, celery, potatoes, onions, tomatoes, green peppers, zucchini, beans, peas, lentils, etc. No meat or meat stock. You may add rice, dehydrated veggies or spices, but use sea salt sparingly. The less you cook the soup, the better. You may have rye wafers with the soup, but not bread or crackers. Make enough for lunch the next day. On the third day, drink orange juice in the morning. Have the rest of the soup for lunch. For dinner, eat whatever vegetarian salads, vegetables or fruit you wish.

What is a healthy diet after the cleanse? I recommend that breakfast be the MC lemonade. In addition, eat a salad every day as well and primarily eat raw fruit, vegetables, seeds, nuts and berries.

Person No. 16
I was going really strong. Today would be my ninth day. I had laxative tea this morning, intending to go forth with my cleanse, maybe even for another week, but I was really hungry when I went to the store to get more syrup and my mom and I bought a lot of fruits for me to dehydrate and eat when I went off the cleanse. (I was going to finish in two days.) However, when I got home I was very hungry and wanted fruit so badly that, even before having orange juice, I had a few green grapes, a few glasses of orange juice, and a bite of apple I was cutting to dehydrate it. I thought it would be okay since I had been on the cleanse, perfectly, for eight days, but my stomach is hurting now even though I've had a lot of water to try to make the stomachache go away. What do I do?

Peter
I've done the exact same thing although it was after ten days. I drank orange juice, ate an orange, a salad, then some almonds, pepperoncini, olives, etc. Within thirty to forty-five minutes, I was sorry because I had pain and an upset stomach. It lasted through the afternoon, but went away gradually that evening.

In my personal experience, the discomfort of breaking the fast the wrong way (eating solid foods too soon) goes away after a day or less. I have heard a second-hand story that I have not been able to verify that much more serious medical consequences are possible if you break your fast without a gradual return to "normal" food.

Person No. 22
Peter, what was wrong with what you ate? Was it that you rushed into a variety of solid foods, or that you just rushed into solid foods period?

Also, someone mentioned earlier that returning to a solid food diet will cause lost weight to return. Is this true? Thanks.

Peter
It was that I rushed into solid foods too fast.

Person No. 14
I am planning on stopping after Day 10. Do you stop everything that you have been having on the fast and just start purely on the juice? How much juice do you drink? Is it breakfast, lunch and dinner or whenever you feel hungry? Can you give me a rough estimate of how many oranges I should be juicing? Can I mix it up a bit and have some grapefruit juice and some orange juice? Many thanks for your help.

Peter
Burroughs says to slowly drink several eight-ounce glasses of fresh orange juice the first two days—with extra water if you want. He goes on to recommend eating vegetable soup in the evening. I have personally found the orange juice too "thick," almost like eating solid food, and instead I used grapefruit juice.

My own experience, having done solid food the first day afterwards and being nauseated, is that you need to be on just juices or you'll feel nauseated. I know of one person who vomited because she went back to solid food the next day.

**Also, be aware that it generally takes two days before most people have BMs again after the MC because there is nothing in the colon to eliminate. If you still are not eliminating, be sure to take probiotics when you return to solid food as probiotics make up 30 percent of the bulk of eliminations. Also, daily green smoothies in the morning promote eliminations due to the fibers in the greens.

Bronchitis, Asthma

Peter
In Germany, Japan and Russia, there are annual medical conferences on the benefits of fasting. The 2001 fasting conference in the Russian Republic of Buryatia heard papers citing the benefits of fasting for treating ten different diseases including asthma, bronchitis, hypertension (high blood pressure), viral lung infections and obesity.

Brushing Your Teeth During the Cleanse

Peter
I see no reason not to brush your teeth. Just don't use toothpaste with artificial flavors, colors, preservatives sweeteners or fluoride. Fluoride is so poisonous that swallowing any more than a pea-sized amount of fluoride toothpaste requires calling a poison control center! (See the warning on your tube of toothpaste.)

During the cleanse, I don't use any toothpaste. Use mint tea to help handle mouth and body odors. By the way, if you are going for a clear, pink tongue as a sign of the cleanse being complete, check your tongue 24 hours after brushing it. What have others done?

Person No. 23
I use IPSAB brand tooth powder. It's a combo of salt, baking soda, prickly ash bark and peppermint oil. It doesn't have all the fillers and other stuff in traditional toothpaste. It also works great on the film on your tongue. I bought it at a health food store.

Candida

Person No. 24
Any feedback on yeast and the MC? Does the maple syrup feed the yeast? Is the cleanse effective for yeast buildup as well as others kinds of toxins? My husband is considering joining us but is concerned about the yeast factor. Thanks. Love and light to all.

Peter
The Master Cleanse is not a guaranteed cure for candida/yeast. 55 percent had no problem before or after. 13 percent had a problem and it was gone after the Master Cleanse. 14 percent didn't have a problem before but did after the Master Clease. 18 percent had a problem before and after. People who have candida before are likely to have it after. The percentages are from a poll that has been running on my website forum for four years that has responses from 180 people.

Person No. 17
My mom has systemic yeast problems and did the cleanse for thirty days. It helped her a lot, but I am afraid I don't have a lot of details about her experience.

Person No. 12
I don't have bad problems with yeast but I have had in the past. I notice it when my diet goes downhill. I have not had any problem with yeast on this fast.

Cayenne Pepper

Peter
Cayenne pepper is such a wonderful herb. I want to share a great web page explaining its virtues. Some people wonder what it does in the Master Cleanse. Here's a good link for more information: www.shirleys-wellness-cafe.com/cayenne.htm.

Person No. 2
OK, I believe you. I am back to putting cayenne pepper in the lemonade. Took Day 4 off from the pepper. Good article, and a must read for anyone making lemonade.

Person No. 16
I don't have any cayenne pepper at the moment. I started the cleanse today. If I don't use the pepper for the first few days, will that affect the results of the cleanse?

Person No. 1
The pepper is very important. Check out the first posting at the top of this topic and go buy the pepper.

If you want great results, don't alter the directions in any way for the cleanse. If you do not have a copy of the Master Cleanse book, buy one. Follow the directions and Good luck!

Person No. 6
I like to use a lot of cayenne pepper. Love the taste. But will overdoing the cayenne alter results? I like to use about 1/2 tsp. per glass. My lemonade is pretty red. Does anyone else out there overdose on the cayenne? If so, what were the results? By the way, everything else is measured out to the T. And I make it two glasses at a time, because one glass doesn't usually satisfy me.

Peter
In *The Master Cleanser*, Stanley Burroughs says to use a tenth of a teaspoon of cayenne or "to taste." So, add all you want. Like you, my son loves it, put in much more than 1/10 teaspoon and had a great result.

● Cayenne pepper acts as the accelerator pedal for the cleanse. It dilates blood vessels, increasing circulation. It feeds the heart, is a great source of Vitamin C, and breaks down mucus & old waste. So, don't skip the cayenne. Also, don't take cayenne in capsules. According to Dr. Richard Schulze, a master herbalist, people who take cayenne capsules do not receive much of the benefit of the cayenne. The nerve endings in the mouth respond almost instantly to send blood throughout the body. This whole process is missed if you take capsules. So, taking cayenne capsules should not be done.

Do not put so much in that you hate the taste of the lemonade and then don't drink it. However, do try to stretch your tolerance of it. Not getting enough cayenne will definitely slow down your cleanse. If you don't like it or are not used to spicy heat, start with a sprinkle of cayenne and gradually increase it as you learn to like it. It is a learned food.

There are three things that will make cayenne hotter: 1) Mixing a whole day's batch and putting cayenne in the drink when you make it. Cayenne gets stronger the longer it sits in the drink. 2) Not shaking or stirring the container before drinking. This is especially true if you work and make several glasses at once. The cayenne will sink to the bottom and the last sips will be very, very hot. 3) There are several strengths of cayenne. The common one sold in supermarkets is usually 30,000 heat units. Health food stores also carry that kind and sometimes another hotter one, African Bird Pepper.

Cheating—Am I Alone?

Person No. 26
Well, I blew it. I ate an orange Sunday morning and ate salad, nuts and olives at a birthday party last night. I feel really bad. I was working very hard, there were a lot of detox symptoms, and I really wanted to get through ten days at least, though I suspect I need more. Anyway, I plan on eating better and trying again in April. Do you have any thoughts? I could sure use some guidance.

Peter
I am assuming that you blew it on Day 2, 3 or 7 as those are usually the ones with the most cravings and detox symptoms. Don't beat yourself up! You took a step forward and did something good for your body. Take pride in the initial step.

Next, check whether you followed the directions in the book exactly. Herbal laxative tea at night, salt water flush every morning, six to twelve ten-ounce drinks of lemonade in the right proportions each day and nothing else except water or perhaps mint tea? If not, you made it tougher on yourself by not eliminating the toxins you are mobilizing. If so, they were just reabsorbed and you had stronger detox symptoms. If that was the case, it was just as well that you went off what you thought was "the Master Cleanse."

Think of cleansing and diet as a lifelong process, not as a one-time event. You don't get a cleansing report card and then go on to other things in life. You learn about you and your body and how the two of you need to get along. Work toward eating more raw vegetables, fruits, nuts, and seeds. Have some fresh juices. Do the Master Cleanse again. The urgent desire to eat something else, anything else, and the desire just to CHEW something are both detox symptoms that will pass with the next elimination or two

Someone mentioned a metallic taste in the mouth. That is also a detox symptom and probably a sign that person has a greater than average amount of toxins to eliminate. In cases such as this, sometimes the full ten days are needed to get the best results.

Person No. 27
Well, I was doing well, but then Day 3 hit, and it was HORRIBLE—just hungry all day, and a massive headache. No specific cravings, just intense hunger no matter how much lemonade I had.

I made it through Day 3, but then on Day 4 (yesterday) I caved, and ate a big piece of bread, which I promptly threw up quite violently within fifteen minutes! They are not kidding when they say you have to ease back into eating. Then I hated myself, felt really sick and had diarrhea for the next five hours or so, so I don't think I absorbed much of the bread! By the evening I felt better and went back on the lemonade.

I decided to just stick with the fast, and am on Day 5 now, feeling great. Or should I really be calling this Day 1, since I cheated yesterday? Come on, 'fess up, has anyone else caved on the cleanse and then continued anyway? I feel really good, have lost seven pounds so far, and I don't just want to give up all the benefits now!

Person No. 17
I have had three dreams on three different nights that I ate food and broke my fast. In all the dreams I was so mad at myself for cheating. Thankfully in my waking state I have not allowed a speck of food to part my lips. However, one day I put my daughter's reheated, leftover pizza to my nose and inhaled deeply for about three minutes. Such ecstasy!

Chemotherapy, Cancer and the Cleanse

Person No. 28
I was diagnosed with ovarian cancer two years ago. I did everything to avoid chemo, but I ended up with no choice. I ended my treatment last June and my prognosis is very good. No cancer cells in my blood tests. I am starting the Master Cleanse tomorrow and looking forward to feeling detoxified. I have heard that detoxifying too fast could stir up too many toxins in the lymph system and be dangerous because my lymph system might not be able to handle it. This cleanse sounds like it is more of a digestive cleanse than a lymph cleanse, but I would like your opinion. Have you had others that needed to detoxify from chemo? Thank you

Peter
I'm glad you asked before leaping into the cleanse. If you have been on chemotherapy less than six months ago, do not do the MC. If you have been on chemotherapy more than six months ago, you should consult a licensed healthcare practitioner before starting the cleanse. Max Gerson, M.D., (www.gerson.org) reported that anywhere between 20–40 percent of each dose of chemotherapy medicine is stored in the body and could be released during detoxification.

Then, if you decide to do the cleanse considering you have had chemo, I would just "stick a toe in the water" and only drink the minimum six drinks of lemonade each day. I would also be sure to take the herbal laxative tea in the evening and drink at least one ounce of water or lemonade for each two pounds of your body weight each day. Be sure to do the salt water flush as given each morning, and take long, soaking hot baths with Epsom salts to draw out toxins. (Do not do this in fluoridated water! Fluoride is more toxic than lead and a serious enzyme inhibitor. Cancer patients and survivors must avoid drinking, bathing or showering in fluoridated water.) The reason for these warnings is that you want to detoxify these residual toxins with a maximum of elimination. So that whatever toxins are loosened/mobilized will be quickly eliminated.

Also, I would immediately discontinue the cleanse if any detox symptoms didn't disappear or lessen with the next day's eliminations or if you are feeling bad on Day 4. Under those circumstances, discontinue the cleanse and use one of the slower methods of detoxification in the Detox Diet Scale. Even then, you may have to eat some cooked rice or bread to slow down the raw food detoxification depending on symptoms. You can always do the Master Cleanse next year, so don't try to push it.

Person No. 68

In August, I was diagnosed with a brain tumor. Most days are filled with headaches, dizziness, nausea, and some visual/balance problems. I've never had regular bowel movements and have always had bloating, gas, and several problems because of that. Since starting the cleanse, all those symptoms have disappeared and I've lost twelve pounds. I'm completely thrilled!! I go back to the neurologist Monday and can't wait to tell him all this.

I plan to eat much healthier, (after breaking the fast appropriately). I have more energy and clarity and feel more like myself. I just wanted to give my "testimony." This has been a godsend.

Chewing Gum

Person No. 29

I started the MC today, 5 Jan 2004. It is very encouraging and motivating to read everyone's questions and comments. I am so excited for my own outcome. I do have a question. Can you chew any kind of gum? Thanks.

Peter

No. Chewing gum consists of five main ingredients: a gum base, sugar, corn syrup, softeners, and flavorings. Some gums include artificial chemicals to sweeten them. These have to be handled by the body as toxins.

Other than a cup of herbal laxative tea in the evening (and optionally one in the morning), a quart of (sea) salt water first thing in the morning, six to twelve drinks of lemon (or lime)ade during the day, occasional mint tea and as much water as you want, nothing else is a part of Stanley Burrough's Master Cleanse regimen. The idea is to give the digestive and elimination organs a rest so they can use their energy to cleanse and rejuvenate.

Cleansing, Other Types

Person No. 1

Is it really necessary for people to do a liver cleanse with olive oil after they complete the Master Cleanse? I am a little hesitant. I was under the impression that the MC was cleaning the liver as well as other internal organs.

Peter

You're correct that the Master Cleanse does also cleanse the liver, kidneys, glands and other parts of the body. People with arthritis have even commented that they noticed joint pain relieved or eliminated.

I have a good friend and business partner who did a ten-day cleanse. He has had a massage every week for several years from his massage therapist. The second week of his cleanse, she told him he had the cleanest liver she'd ever observed. She also said she's never seen anyone's body change so much for the better in her professional life.

I'd be very interested in feedback from people that do another kind of cleanse after the Master Cleanse to see if they notice any difference.

Person No. 1

Peter, Thank you so very much for this website!

Your responses to my questions and the feedback from others have been very helpful. This is Day 10 of the MC for me and my tongue is very pink and my breath smells good! I have decided to extend my fast a few more days to see if I will have any additional effects/benefits.

Question: Is it safe to say that with an extended MC fast at some point in time the body will start eliminating all mucus and nothing else?

Peter

Definitely, although the waste does come off in layers.

When I did my first cleanse (twenty days), I had just bright yellow (bile?) liquid after the eighth day. However, on the seventeenth day, I passed some semi-solid waste!

I'm on Day 16 of my third cleanse and for the first ten days, I had some semi-solid material every day. It's quite amazing how much stuff there is inside a person.

Cold, Feeling

Person No. 12

I am cold all day long and all night. I am trying to stay warm. I have turned up the heat, put on more clothes etc. I have been getting the chills ever since I started this cleanse. I sure hope this is a common side effect. The weather here in Atlanta goes up and down, some days colder than others. Even when I'm inside I'm cold. My hands, feet and nose are the coldest! Anyone else?

Person No. 8

Yea, I don't know why Peter couldn't have suggested doing this in July when the chills would feel good! Anyway, the pepper is supposed to help with the chills, so if you can add more pepper it might help. We also heated up the lemonade one day just because we were so cold. You don't get as much benefit from it but it felt good.

Person No. 13

I was a bit cold my first couple days. Now as of my sixth day I don't seem to be having that problem anymore.

Person No. 6

Today is Day 10 for me! And I have to say that I have had the chills from Day 1 until today. Glad to know it's not just me. But I have been freezing throughout the entire cleanse! Fleece is my friend!

Peter

Any sort of fasting lowers metabolism and that means the body is colder. The Master Cleanse fits right in there. By the way, the idea that you want to have fast metabolism so you can eat a lot has a darker side. As detailed by Joel Fuhrman, M.D. in his book *Eat to Live*, a slower metabolism can lead to extended lifespan if you eat the right (vegetarian) foods.

As for July instead of January, that's a great idea. Actually, I was planning to promote Master Cleanses quarterly, but seeing all the great results people are getting, I think I will just promote cleanses whenever someone is ready.

Colonics

Person No.10

Has anyone done a colonic or are we cleansing our colons well enough? I hate the thought of those things but really want to be "cleaned out!"

Also, does this cleanse clean the liver or should I do a liver cleanse next?

Thanks for any input you can offer.

Peter

I have done colonics before the first Master Cleanse and done an herbal cleanse after the first MC as well to see the difference. I have found the

Master Cleanse is the best for me and I have no need for colonics. Others I've talked to like colonics and have done them after the Master Cleanse.

I think it comes back to the waste accumulating in layers in the colon. There are many years of waste in most people's colons and that takes several Master Cleanses or several colonics. I would not do colonics while on the Master Cleanse, though.

Although Burroughs warns against colonics and says they only clean out the last few feet of the colon (good point), the choice to use them is a personal one. The one thing I know with great certainty is that people's bodies are different and respond differently to treatment.

With regard to needing other cleanses after this one, see the topic "Cleansing, Other Types" above.

● Cramping

Person No. 67
For those who suffer from unexplainable cramping, here's something to try. After reading the website on the benefits of cayenne pepper, I tried something and it worked immediately. I took a little more than one-half teaspoon of cayenne, put it on the back of my tongue, and took a drink of lemonade. The cramping stopped instantly! I also had to eliminate immediately afterwards. It was like a miracle. It also worked with menstruation cramps.

Cravings

Person No. 30
I'm on the fifth day of my first MC. I've had this craving for milk—a cold, tall glass of milk—for the last three days. I've always been a milk drinker, but lately, I wasn't drinking as much. But now, I'm really craving it. Is this normal? It doesn't help because my son is a huge milk drinker too and our fridge is stocked with two whole gallons of milk! I wonder if I'll last another five days.

Person No. 21
Hi Person No.30: I'm on my fifth day too. I've craved Thai food since the beginning of the fast. I think the lemon along with the cayenne is reminding me of it. From what I've read cravings are pretty normal with this fast. You're half way there! Don't give in now. You can do it.

Person No. 1

It has been said that when you are having cravings your body is removing those toxins from your body and that the cravings will go away after your morning BMs.

This is Day 8 for me. I feel really great. Whatever mild cravings I had were gone by the evening hours of Day 5. Whatever you do, do not quit! You have completed the hardest part of the fast. Good luck!

Person No. 30

Thanks for the responses! You were right, my cravings have subsided.

Person No. 11

Hi everyone! Today is Day 3 for me on my first MC. I tried to start Monday but by dinnertime I gave in and ate! So, I started over. The first two days were really tough with the cravings. So, I had a cup of organic veggie broth each day! I wonder how badly that will impact my detoxing. I almost quit last night because we had family over for dinner and the smell of the food drove me insane! Today I woke up feeling okay. Anyway, I am glad I found this forum. Knowing that other people feel my "pain" will help me get through this. Good luck, everyone!

Peter

**The first two days are the worst and trying to do it for the first time with family over and them cooking is heroic! Unfortunately, drinking veggie broth will only prolong the cravings and detox symptoms. Whatever the body is detoxing and eliminating is what you're craving. If you keep putting stuff in, it will continuously be eliminated and thus keep the cravings going. You want to avoid that.

Person No. 11

Thanks for the info, Peter. I will resist the temptation to drink the veggie broth! It's tough to do this, especially when my husband is crunching into an oooh-soo-delicious-sounding grilled cheese sandwich! Ah, this is so hard! Thank goodness I found this forum!

Daily Experiences

Person No. 1

This is Day 8 for me. I feel really good. No food cravings. Lots of energy. My tongue is clearing and my breath/mouth feels/smells good. My skin looks really good. The white portion of my eyes looks whiter than usual. If I feel okay at Day 10, I may extend my fast to fourteen days, but I'll take it one day at a time. I have not felt this great in years. I have passed *The Master Cleanser* book to a number of friends.

Person No. 11

I am on Day 4. I didn't wake up with huge cravings—and seeing a cup of coffee and a jar of peanut butter didn't drive me to seizures either! I feel a little icky, I woke up and my body just sort of ached

Interesting to note: last summer I got ringworm on my leg from a puppy my brother adopted from the Humane Society. I cured my leg by using essential oils and it went away, except I had a dark patch on my skin where I had it. On Day 2 of my cleanse, I was out shoveling snow (we got hit hard in Toronto this week). I thought I got frostbite because my leg was feeling just like I had burned it on the ringworm area. This lasted about two days. Today I woke up, no pain, and more importantly, no more dark patch of skin! Could this be part of the whole detox thing? I am feeling so happy! It's hard to explain: aside from the physical symptoms, this is turning out to be a very spiritual thing. I hope to be able to keep the positive attitude and make my goal of ten days! I hope you are all achieving great milestones as well! Hang in there and don't give up!

Person No. 11

I forgot to add that I stepped on the scale this morning and weighed five pounds less!!!

Person No. 10

Day 9, tongue is almost pink (actually was yesterday), short term memory sucks! Today I feel tired, possibly because it is Saturday so I am allowing it. Generally feel great, can move all joints freely and that is awesome!

I have lost thirteen pounds, but have done this many times before and do not do this for weight loss. I do it to cleanse and to return to good eating habits. However, I do want to lose at least seven more pounds.

Person No. 21

This is my first MC. I'm on Day 7 and feeling great. My tongue is already turning pink. It isn't perfectly pink but it is definitely clearing. I've been very generous with the cayenne in my lemonade. I wonder if that is helping to move things along. I love the taste of it. My sense of smell has greatly increased. My hubby and I took our boys to the Air and Space Museum yesterday and everywhere I turned I smelled halitosis.

I keep reading online about liver and parasite cleanses and wonder if I need that or not.

Peter

Burroughs says the Master Cleanse will cleanse all the organs and glands including the kidneys and liver. From experience, I know that the Master Cleanse handles parasites. Other nutritional, natural healers, including Norman Walker, have said parasites require waste accumulations in order to find good breeding grounds. So it makes sense that the Master Cleanse also handles parasites.

Person No. 8

Unfortunately, I had to get off of the cleanse on Day 6. I was just too hungry and getting hungrier all of the time, no matter how much lemonade or water I had. The first four days were fine and then I started getting hungry—very hungry. My husband just finished Day 10 and feels good. He had to stop the tea and the salt water for a couple of days because of work, but even though he did, he eliminated today. He said it was real black and really stunk. Good sign. He is getting rid of a lot of old toxins. He is shooting to go to twenty days. I don't really get cravings for SAD (Standard American Diet) foods but he does. We are hoping the cleanse will take care of those cravings.

Person No. 6

I am on Day 1. I chose to quit smoking and do the cleanse at the same time and I have never experienced a more pleasant experience quitting smoking. I hardly think of smoking at all because I've had these weird food cravings since last night in spurts. I'd crave certain foods so bad, I could smell them. Give me a choice between a cigarette and a Whopper and the Whopper wins! At any rate, it's just after 1:30 p.m. I've just polished off my third glass of lemonade. And I've had five BMs today, which left me really tired and lethargic for about an hour. And now I'm fine and, surprisingly, not hungry. I want to satiate some weird taste bud war going on in my mouth. Other than the few cramps I had this morning, my stomach is fine.

Person No. 31

I am on Day 4. This is my second attempt at MC. I stopped the first time at Day 3 because of my food cravings. For the past year, I have disciplined myself to stay away from certain foods so that makes this MC much easier. Instead of wanting a burger, I really just want a big salad. My stomach starts to cramp when I need to eliminate some toxins and then I go to the bathroom and they go away. I'm not really hungry at all and I have sufficient energy for the day's activities.

Person No. 11
**I am experiencing the whole heightened sense of smell, too. I had a friend come over and he smelled like snot! He has good hygiene and I was baffled by this new thing. I couldn't bear to be too close to him because I could just smell this "congestion" smell emanating from him. I went to the mall and it was like hitting a brick wall. It smelled AWFUL!

Person No. 6
I'm on Day 2 of the cleanse. I was doing soooo well today up until an hour ago when I had to help my little one prepare a tasty sandwich for herself.

I did offer up a few new rules in my household, which may benefit others living with children.

Rule #1—No eating in the car!

Rule #2—No eating around mommy for first few days of the cleanse!

Rule #3—Mommy will not be cooking during the cleanse. (To supplement this rule, we went grocery shopping and stockpiled on favorite microwavable dinners, fresh fruits, veggies and goodies to make tasty sandwiches.) Mom's taking a break from cooking for a while.

In the long run, it's beneficial all around, because in my household we were never healthy eaters and this cleanse gives me the time to reflect on how to slowly but surely change bad eating habits to good eating habits.

Person No. 24
Hi folks. Day 3 for me. I feel much better than I did. Lots of muscle aches and lower back pain today. The first day I was really sick like the flu, with nightmares and anxiety the first night. Then my vertebrae started adjusting—just like early pregnancy! It's like everything is loose again. I felt much better yesterday, more bored than sick (also detox symptoms I hear) and today my body aches are the rule of the morning. I can't wait to see what freedom comes after these aches pass! I am really committed to ten days minimum. This fast has been too long in coming. I tried the MC four years ago and only made it a couple days and I have had adult acne ever since. My skin is already clearing up by Day 3. Think of all the time, grief and money I could have saved by just cleansing and changing my diet!! Have a great day!

Person No. 8

My husband is just finishing up Day 14. He is not hungry, just missing being able to chew food. Energy level normal. Since we eat 90 percent raw, he already is in pretty good shape. He has lost fifteen pounds so far. His tongue is just starting to look a little better. Not so coated. His breath is starting to smell not quite so bad. Boy, was that awful for awhile. He's shooting to go twenty days or less if his tongue turns pink first. Even though I didn't make it all ten days (only six since I kept getting hungrier and hungrier) I find that I am eating less and sleeping less with the same amount of energy I had before. So, all of you people just starting, hang in there. You won't regret it.

Person No. 12

Hi. I started Saturday morning, so today is my third day. The hardest part for me was Day 1 and 2.

One word of advice, don't announce the cleanse to every person you meet to feed any ego that you may have or excitement to tell all. Don't argue with the uneducated. Don't try to convince other people until you educate yourself. Don't set yourself up for failure or negative feedback. I have only let a few close friends in on my great adventure. So far, so good! Best of luck to all and to all a spicy lemonade! Talk atcha soon.

Person No. 11

I actually prepared dinner tonight for my husband and daughter. While I acknowledge the fact that it would be nice to taste what I made, I was able to NOT TAKE A SINGLE NIBBLE! How's that for self-restraint?

Person No. 3

I am on Day 7. I can't believe I have made it this far. I will say that today is the first day I have had cravings of any kind. I am really hungry today and I had a lot of abdominal cramping. I am still debating whether to go twenty days. A part of me says go for it and a part of me says I miss food, especially when you go out to dinner with friends and family and you are the only one not eating. That happened four times this weekend!

Person No. 32

Today is Day 8 for me. So far today has been the best day. I feel serene, at peace. My thinking is shifting. It's really wonderful. I'm still a little tired in the evening, but I suppose that is to be expected. Or, if Peter is right, maybe tomorrow I won't be tired anymore. Hope so!

Person No. 16

Today would have been my ninth day but I had to quit because I was getting a little restless, but up until today I have been very into the MC, very happy, a lot of energy. But I'm glad today to get some fruit.

Peter

"Restlessness" is just another detox symptom, but I'm glad you had a good cleanse. When you feel like it, do another Master Cleanse. They just get easier and better.

Person No. 33

Day 9: Day 10 will begin once I go to bed. I have a rash on my face. I have gone through moments of feeling great, mentally fresh and feelings of exuberance. I really would like to go to Day 20. My goal is to continue until my face has cleared up. For me the bumps on my face are a detox symptom. My skin has always been very clear.

Person No. 18

I'm on Day 8 and I feel fantastic. I'm quite proud of myself and have even recruited about five others to do the cleanse. I had to call and encourage my sister and her husband last night. It was their first day and although they said it was rough they both seemed determined. I had a larger than usual BM this morning after a day of heavy cayenne pepper in the lemonade. All in all, life is good.

Person No. 18

I'm on Day 9 and I plan to go past the ten-day mark and shoot for at least fourteen. I was utterly amazed this morning at how much stuff came out. I concluded that the tea and salt water had really broken up a lot of my old intestinal waste. I definitely shed some layers this morning. If I can make it thru Superbowl weekend (it's here in Houston where I live) and all the festivities, then I think that twenty days might really be possible for me. That would be awesome for my first cleanse.

Person No. 33

I am on Day 13. My husband stopped on Day 11. I was feeling great. But, last night I began to have mucus. It surprised me somewhat because I thought the cleansing was done. I also have this annoying rash on my face. I thought that it was getting better but it seems to be moving about my face. If anyone has any idea what it may be from let me know. I thought maybe it was toxins, but now I don't know. I am committed to stay on the lemonade drink until the rash is gone. My plan is to stay until Day 20.

Peter

Some of the by-products of meat digestion are toxins in addition to which, the body treats artificial colors, flavors and preservatives, alcohol, soda, beer, wine, tobacco and drugs as though they are poisons. To the many people who are lactose intolerant, dairy has the same toxic effect. It attempts to handle this condition by sending white blood cells (leukocytes). It also creates a layer of mucus in the colon to protect the body from absorbing these poisons directly into the blood stream.

As you release toxins on the cleanse, it is quite probable that the body is creating mucus to attempt handle the newly released toxins before they are eliminated. The handling, of course, would be to continue the cleanse or do another when time permits to eliminate more of the toxins.

The rash is also probably a result of the detox. That it is moving around on your face shows that change is happening. Detoxing is a change. We want that.

A friend had a history of hemorrhoids. On the second day of the cleanse (just three weeks ago) he got bleeding hemorrhoids, but they were not as painful as before. A few days later they went away. He feels they will never come back as long as he keeps his diet relatively clean.

Day 1

Person No. 13

First day on the cleanse. I have done a couple of fasts before, but not really anything close to this. The first fast I did only lasted a couple of days. I was drinking fresh veggie and fruit juice, but I became violently ill on the third day—vomiting and diarrhea. I don't believe this was due to the detox because I have been a raw vegan—with some cheating—for about seven months and I went through a bad detox period when I started as a vegan. I think what happened was that I let my veggie juice sit too long.

The second fast I did was six days, but it wasn't really complete because I ended up using some processed juices due to work / laziness. This did me some good but I have a feeling this fast will be much better.

I had initially planned to do this Master Cleanse for fourteen days, but I keep reading here that twenty days is optimal. So, I will try to make it for the twenty.

I have not done a salt flush yet. I am using the laxative tea so far, but I think I will try a salt flush tomorrow. I have yet to eliminate and don't know how much waste to expect, especially since I have been a raw foodist and things normally move through me very quickly. The last fast I did, I was still eliminating five days into it. That's a ton of backup. Now I tend to think I don't have a lot of backup, but then again I was on the SAD (Standard American Diet) for 22 years. There is no telling what's in there.

If there are any other short-term raw foodists here who have done this cleanse, I'd be curious to know how it affected you in general and how much waste you expelled/how quickly. Otherwise, I hope to stay positive and have no major problems doing this. I will post sometimes to update on my progress.

Person No. 27
This is my first day on the fast too, so I thought I would offer you support since I will need it myself! We are polar opposites as far as our normal diets. I have never even been a vegetarian, much less raw vegan. I am curious as to what sort of different results this fast will have on each of us. I was afraid I would be terribly hungry, but I have not been too hungry. Good luck!

Person No. 13
Thanks. Good luck to you too. My fast is either going really well or really bad depending on how I look at it. I'm in a lot of pain from burning BMs.

Peter
My first twenty-day Master Cleanse was after six months of a 100 percent raw vegetable/fruit/nut/seed diet. I had already lost over thirty pounds on that diet and proceeded to lose another twenty on the Master Cleanse. I had burning BMs for four or five days and was amazed at all I had to get out.

I read your post, Person No.13, and given the reaction you are having now with the burning pain, I'd say you probably started a serious detox on your juice cleanse rather than a reaction from letting the veggie juice "sit too long."

● I'm always quite surprised by who ends up having severe detox symptoms on the cleanse. Sometimes it's medications they took and/or food they ate long before their current diet that caused the symptoms.

The solution is to emphasize the elimination part of the Master Cleanse. Drink lots of lemonade and the laxative tea, do the salt water flush and continue. If it gets really bad, discontinue the cleanse and eat raw fruits and vegetables to detox more slowly. You can always do the cleanse again later.

Person No. 13
Yes, my former habits explain a lot about the pain. Thanks.

Day 3—Feeling Good

Person No. 14
Just wanted to say that I have reached Day 3 and am feeling surprisingly good. Day 1 and 2 were quite hard. Although I don't like to quit anything, last night I was tempted to cut this thing short. Today I feel very excited, enthusiastic and optimistic about everything. So my advice to anyone on Day 1 or 2 is just to get through it. It seems much better after those two hard days. The SWF (salt water flush) is awful, but I would say it is really important to do it. The results are fantastic. Good luck to everyone who is cleansing. It's a really good thing to do.

Person No. 12
Good for you. I agree. Day 1-3 were the worst for me. I started on a Saturday surrounded by kids and my hubby eating crap in front of me. Crap that I usually eat!! I am on Day 5 and this is my first MC. I have not had a solid movement yet, but I am looking forward to it. It's crazy but good that we can talk about our daily eliminations to each other.

This website helps me with support no one else understands! I can say though, my hubby has been supportive and proud of me. Good luck to you. Have you done this before? My goal is fourteen days. Ending my MC on January 30th unless I feel detoxified before that. Heck, I may keep going if need be!

Person No. 14
Thanks for all your lovely words of encouragement. This is my first MC. I became a raw foodist last August and that has been great. Christmas broke my willpower and I ate so much crap it was unreal. I took a look at myself a couple of weeks ago and I looked bad. My skin had broken out. I had cold sores and I felt terrible. So, I thought I needed a good

clean out, which is why I am doing this. Hopefully, it will put me on the straight and narrow again and I can go back to eating all my lovely raw food again. It's been hard for me cooking and watching my husband and two kids eat food. I think the masochist in me is making me cook all the foods that I really love. Fortunately, I have iron willpower and I won't give up. I am going to keep going for the ten days then I will see how I feel and maybe go a bit longer. It seems a shame to get so far and then stop when you know you need to detox a bit more. So who knows, I'll see how I feel next week. Lovely to talk to you and thanks for all your kind words.

Person No. 13
This is my third day too and while I am having some burning still, I feel ten times better than I did the past two days. In addition to pain, I also had so many toxins floating about that I was completely disoriented and couldn't concentrate on anything. I also slept a whole lot, but this is probably a good thing. I'm going to continue to twenty days. This is perfect because I will be ending on Saturday, Feb. 7th, then I can do fruit juice and some oranges on Sunday, and have my first big salad again on that Monday. Oh, how I look forward to that salad.

It's amazing how fast you start to see your face change after you cheat on your raw diet, isn't it? You get all puffy and pale, and lose the glow. The good thing is that you get it right back when you go back to 100 percent raw. I cheated for about a month straight on my raw diet, and boy did I look and feel bad.

I can't say I am perfect. I cheat every now and then, but the rewards never add up. It only makes me feel bad and remember why I went raw to begin with. Good luck!

Person No. 14
You are so right about the face. I've just been to the bathroom and as I turned round—I have a big mirror—I have just this minute thought to myself how much better my face is looking–not quite so old somehow. How long have you been raw? At times I find it quite a challenge. Especially if I'm facing some stress—that old thing of reaching for food when you're under stress. Overall though I love how it makes me look and feel and it makes so much sense. It's nice to talk to someone else who has found raw food. I am the only person where I live who is into it. I think most people think I'm a little extreme. So, it's great to find a like-minded person. I think we may have strayed from the topic of the Master Cleanse, but I guess it's sort of related. Good luck on Day 4 and on reaching your goals.

Person No. 13

I have been raw for almost eight months—really seven because I cheated almost every day for one entire month. I do cheat occasionally, and yes it is normally in times of stress, going back to old comforts, etc. Sometimes I allow myself to cheat because I feel I deserve it, which is silly because I'm saying that I deserve to mess my body up. I also know that I recover fast and when I do cheat, I don't cheat badly. I usually only eat cooked veggies. Bread and rice make me horribly ill.

Yes, it is looked upon as extreme and I am the only person here as well who is raw or even vegan. However I have a couple of friends online who give me support and that helps. Otherwise, I just know that this is the best thing to do—the only thing that makes sense and gives you proper nourishment. It's simple. It's called nature, but most people are so conditioned from birth that this natural way of eating seems totally preposterous to them. I guess we are getting on a different topic.

I try my best and generally feel great. I know I'll feel even better after I do this cleanse. I'm so glad this bulletin board is here. It helps a lot to keep me going because this thing is no picnic, but I know it will be worth it in the end.

Day 5

Person No. 1

This is Day 5 for me. As I mentioned previously, I had a sore throat for the past day and a half and itchy inner ears. Well, IT'S ALL GONE AWAY! I just have a runny nose (clear mucus)—no thick stuff yet. I guess I was pretty toxic after all. This is my first time doing the MC. I am convinced that the MC is the right thing to do for overall good body health. I will do this the recommended three to four times a year for life. I will also modify my diet. I have asthma so I have concerns as to what detox symptoms I will experience as a result of it while on the MC.

Person No. 10

Day 5 for me too and I feel great. I have done this so many times and have never felt as good as when I am on the cleanse. It was as if my body had seized up and is now releasing and I can move freely again. I am going to continue until my tongue is pink (although this time it isn't as bad as other times when it got a thick yellow coating).

I am not doing the salt water flush as the last couple of times I gagged but instead am drinking laxative tea night and morning and I am definitely "flushing."

Person No. 34
Today is Day 7 for me. The first four days were very good—I felt good. Then on Day 5 I started to feel really horrible with stomachaches and stuff. I continued the cleanse and on Day 6 the symptoms started to go away. Now, I'm feeling a lot better. The good things I've noticed so far are my face is clearing up, I feel much more energized, my plugged left ear cleared up and my sinus infection went away! I was planning to go the ten days but I might go a little longer to fully clear up my tongue. It was the most white yesterday but today it's less. So, we'll see.

Day 10!

Person No. 21
I'm on my tenth day of the MC and I think I'm going to keep on going. It is kind of funny, when I started I was determined to make ten days, but felt it would be really hard. I was even planning what kind of food I would treat myself to when I was done (Thai Food). Now, I really feel the need to get rid of more toxins. I woke up this morning with a lot of nasal mucus. I think this is going to be a big detox day and I really don't think I should end the fast that way. I want to be completely clear. I've had so many improvements in my health along the way. I have no need for my asthma or allergy meds. My eczema is clearing and I have no acne. I'm no longer eating when I'm confronted with stressful situations. So onward I must go. Thanks for all of your help everyone.

Peter
Wow, Person No. 21, you're inspiring! I can identify with all that. I won't quit on a detox day and I like Thai food when I'm not eating raw.

Person No. 11
Hi everyone! It is now Day 10 for me and I am sooo excited! I can't believe I made it through. My tongue is not completely pink yet. I had thought about extending the fast, but since it is my first time, I will be a wimp and finish it today. Yes, I do miss food a lot! I am really looking forward to that veggie salad or soup. I lost a total of nine pounds. I was a little disappointed that it wasn't more but realistically, I am 5'1" and down to 106 pounds. So, any more probably wouldn't be healthy. I would love to hit the 99-100 pound mark though. Ah, the college days! Maybe if I extend the fast I would lose more, but I want to keep the reason for the fast in perspective and it was never to lose weight to begin with. I would like to know from people who have done this before, did they gain all the weight back? How long did it take? I am

curious and a little scared. I am attached to my rib count now! Anyway, thanks for all the support everyone, best of luck on the MC and I will probably be back in a few months to do it all over again!

Peter

You raise a good question about regaining the weight. I lost a little more than twenty pounds on my first twenty-day cleanse. I then stayed on mostly raw veggies/fruit/nuts/seeds with occasional forays into ribs, ice cream and the bad stuff for fun. I'd say I was about 90–95 percent raw. I then did two more ten-day cleanses just because I liked them. By then it was a year later and my weight was about the same as when I finished the first cleanse. Before the first cleanse, I ate a 100 percent raw veggie, etc. diet for six months and lost 32 pounds! None of that has come back.

It's all about what you eat. If you eat the "bad stuff," which the body sees as toxins, the body will protect itself by making mucus to line the digestive tract and store the toxins in the body fat. Eat junk and get fat. If you eat real food, food with nutritive value, you will lose to an ideal weight and not gain it back at all. There you go: total control of your weight and health.

Person No. 12

I just wanted to say thanks to everyone (especially Peter) for all the advice and support. I have entered into Day 10 and I am going for Day 14! I figure I'm already here and I have no more weekends to get through. I might as well.

I have seen great results. For everyone out there doubting it or wanting to quit, hold out! Not only is it a great test of will, it is overall the best feeling of good health you'll ever experience! Your sense of food appreciation grows tremendously and self discipline is at its highest. Respect for your body (temple) is found quickly. We are what we eat— how true, how true. Thanks again. God bless.

Person No. 10

Thank you to everyone for your words of encouragement, knowledge and shared experiences. I am now on Day 11 and I feel terrific! I am quitting today but staying on broth for ten days. I would like to lose a few more pounds and really get committed to my health. I don't trust that if I return to normal eating today I will "behave," so the broth option is great for me.

My skin is so clear and glowing. I've lost fifteen pounds. I am at peace and proud of myself! I have done this at least ten times before and this was the easiest ever. Good health and happiness to you all for 2004 and beyond.

Diabetics, Special Instructions

Peter

I have had a number of people with diabetes ask about doing the Master Cleanse. In *Healing for the Age of Enlightenment*, Burroughs instructs diabetics to use only a bare tablespoon of molasses in the lemonade at first while decreasing the amount of insulin slightly. Then each day gradually increase the amount of molasses while decreasing the amount of insulin, regularly checking the sugar level in the urine and blood to ensure it is within normal range. When you reach two tablespoons of molasses and the insulin has been eliminated, switch to two tablespoons of organic Grade B maple syrup instead of molasses. Upon completing the Master Cleanse, a diet of fresh raw vegetables, nuts, seeds and fruits is recommended as Burroughs describes diabetes as the result of nutritional deficiencies due to a white sugar and white flour diet. Before following these instructions you should consult with your licensed healthcare practitioner.

Diarrhea

Person No. 35

I'm starting my second day of the MC. Yesterday went fine and I drank the tea before bed. I had a restless night of sleep as my tummy was "rumbly" all night. I could only get down one-half the salt water this morning, so I am making more laxative tea. I already have diarrhea. Is this normal? Should I drink more tea?

Peter

Is it actually diarrhea or just four or five watery bowel movements from the salt water? Diarrhea lasts all day. The salt water flush only produces eliminations for an hour or so starting thirty to sixty minutes after you drink the salt water. If it is really diarrhea, discontinue the laxative tea and salt water until the diarrhea is gone. Your body is getting rid of wastes.

Person No. 35

Unfortunately it's the real deal along with incredible cramping. So, are you saying I should stop the laxative tea till the diarrhea subsides? I haven't been able to find the book locally. I am going to order it today. In the meantime, I really appreciate the bulletin board to answer questions. Today is much more challenging than yesterday. But I just kept reminding myself that you said the symptoms will most likely subside with the next morning's flush. Thanks for the encouragement.

Peter
If the diarrhea continues for more than three days, discontinue the cleanse. Eating grated raw apples or cooked white rice generally stops diarrhea. If that doesn't stop it, you should see a licensed healthcare practitioner since diarrhea can be serious if it continues for a long time.

Emotional Detox?

Person No. 35
Hi Everyone. It sure helps to read how everyone is doing. I am just about through Day 4 and, like many of you, I'm wondering if I'll make it. My hunger comes and goes, same with the cravings. I seem to be craving things I don't normally eat, which I find comical: pizza, bratwurst, a ham and cheese sandwich.

Day 2 was a physical detox day for me and today, Day 4, has felt like an emotional detox. Has anyone else experienced an "emotional detox?" I had a dream just before I woke up that triggered the various fears I've been carrying around for weeks. They all surfaced en masse today and I found I just had to face them and deal with them. I'm doing better this evening.

As far as elimination goes, the only thing I'm eliminating is bile. I'm on my third day of diarrhea and not doing the salt water or the laxative tea. Is anyone else having this issue? Thanks for this site, everyone.

Peter
I have had plenty of "emotional detox days" and so have others. One lady had a dream that resolved an emotional problem she had had for years. Another gained a closer relationship with God. Not everyone has these. What I found on my twenty-day cleanse was that the second ten days for me were learning to handle problems without turning to food. In addition to that valuable lesson, I also gained a much more pleasant and even-tempered disposition. I think that these benefits are perhaps the reasons many religions and Indian tribes use fasts to help the spiritual nature of man.

Regarding the diarrhea, your body is getting rid of wastes. As long as it doesn't continue for more than four or five days, I'd continue. If it goes on beyond that, you should probably discontinue the cleanse. If that doesn't stop it, you should see a health professional. Diarrhea can be serious if it continues for a long time.

Person No. 12
Some may call it an emotional detox. I call it a spiritual break-through.

Emotional Eating

Peter
One benefit I gained from my twenty-day cleanse was the ability to face stress without handling it with food.

Exercise, Running, and Weights

Peter
There are two types of exercise: Those that strengthen the heart and circulation (aerobic) and those that build muscle. Running, jogging, and bicycling are examples of aerobic exercise. This type of exercise is very compatible with the Master Cleanse. In fact, most people report being able to do better for longer periods while on the MC, with the occasional detox day—usually Days 2, 3, 7, 14—where you may feel tired. But in general most people have much more energy. Muscle building, however, is not compatible with the Master Cleanse as there is no protein with which to rebuild muscles. Just in case you are worried about going without protein for ten, twenty or more days, Joel Fuhrman, M.D., makes the point in his book, *Fasting—and Eating—for Health*, that the average non-overweight person has enough nutrient reserves to fast for at least forty days.

Friends and Family

Peter
Don't announce the cleanse to every person you meet. Don't argue with the uneducated. Don't try to convince other people. Don't set yourself up for failure or negative feedback. Tell those close friends who you know will support you on your great adventure.

Hair Loss

Peter

Very rarely (perhaps 1 out of 500 or so), a woman (I have never heard it happening to a man) temporarily loses more hair than usual after a cleanse. In every case, their hair has grown back. In the two cases I checked into personally, both women had done cleanses once a month for at least three months in a row. In each case taking extra vitamins, minerals and healthy food produced new, healthy hair. I have heard it said that it results from lack of protein, but this doesn't make sense as what about the other 499 who went without protein for as many or more days. I believe it may result from a lack of alkaline mineral reserves (calcium, magnesium, potassium and sodium) due to too many cleanses too close together. The toxins that are being detoxified are acids and need to be neutralized by the alkaline minerals mentioned above. This is why I recommend waiting at least three months between cleanses. Strangely, I have never heard of anyone losing hair regardless of how long their cleanse went. I have heard from people who have gone forty and even sixty-eight days. It only seems to occur if a person does monthly Master Cleanses for at least three months in a row.

Headaches on the Cleanse

Peter

Having talked to perhaps six or eight people who experienced headaches on the first few days of the cleanse, I want to pass on what I've learned.

Coming off a heavy caffeine habit (coffee, sodas, or tea) on the cleanse occasionally causes headaches even in people who eat healthy food and are otherwise in good shape. If you are coming off caffeine, be sure to have six to twelve drinks of the lemonade each day along with plenty of water to wash out the toxins. In addition, be sure to follow the instructions on the salt water flush and the laxative tea. You want to eliminate as many of the toxins as fast as you can. Most important of all, recognize that the headaches are detox symptoms from quitting a caffeine addiction. They usually go away in one or two days. The most I have heard of are four days. Persist.

Person No. 34

I used to drink one to two cups of coffee daily before I did the cleanse the first time. The first day of the cleanse that time, I had the worst headache I think I've ever had. By the second day it was just barely there and by the third it was completely gone. I never returned to a daily ritual of a morning coffee since the first cleanse, so when I started the cleanse the second time I had no headache at all this time.

Person No. 2

I can relate to the headache. I've concluded it was my coffee addiction. I did a MC in May and didn't have the headaches that I did this time, but I started drinking coffee in September and was having two or more cups a day with about four or more cups of Earl Grey tea. I definitely feel it was coffee. I craved coffee the first three days. Woke up Day 4, no craving and no headache.

Check your tongue. You'll see how white it is to go with the headache. Hang in there—my headache went away totally by Day 4. Make sure you are getting lots of lemonade and water. My error was drinking only four lemonades. Still can't get beyond that, but made up with water.

Person No. 36

This will be the first MC fast for my spouse and me. She had a question regarding headaches. She has to take something every day for headaches, usually Sudafed, or the headache will go into a migraine. She is concerned that when we start the fast the headaches will become unbearable. What should she do?

Peter

When she does the cleanse, she must keep in all the elimination steps: herbal laxative tea, salt water flush, lots of lemonade (six to twelve ten-ounce drinks a day) and plenty of water. If the headaches get to be too bad, she can take her headache medicine for a day or two.

Health—Attitudes About

Peter

1. Each person is responsible for her or his own health.

2. It is wise for a person to learn how to maintain and/or improve their health.

3. Valuable knowledge is available if you take the time to look for it and are willing to determine for yourself whether any knowledge presented is true or false.

4. Each person's body is potentially different. For example, most people find penicillin valuable for killing bacteria. Some people are allergic and might die from it.

5. Diagnosis or advice from a health professional is frequently essential, but each person is responsible to determine if it is true or not for his or her own body and whether to follow the treatment.

6. You must use your own good judgment and experience if you decide to apply the knowledge in my book or on my website or forum. Do not accept it blindly. This may mean consulting a licensed healthcare practitioner.

Hemorrhoids

Peter

A friend had a history of hemorrhoids. On the second day of the cleanse he got bleeding hemorrhoids, but they were not as painful as before. A few days later they went away. He feels they will never come back as long as he keeps his diet relatively clean.

High Blood Pressure

Peter

Fasting is known to reduce high blood pressure. In fact, there is a scientific study done on 174 people with high blood pressure. After a ten-day water fast, everyone on medication was able to come off it. In Germany, Japan and Russia, there are annual medical conferences on the benefits of fasting. The 2001 Russian conference heard papers citing the benefits of fasting for treating ten different diseases including asthma, bronchitis, hypertension (high blood pressure), viral lung infections and obesity.

Please note if you are on high blood pressure medications you may need to have the dosage reduced or you will experience a double whammy: the cleanse reducing blood pressure and the meds.

Regardless of whether you are on meds or not, stand up or sit up slowly. You may be light-headed from the toxins for your first few cleanses.

Honey vs. Maple Syrup

Person No. 69

Can honey be substituted for maple syrup?

Peter

Burroughs says never use honey internally. It is predigested by bees and goes directly into the blood stream—like alcohol—spiking blood sugar and prompting the body to reduce it by secreting insulin, which lowers the blood sugar, which promotes depression.

I wouldn't go as far as to say never to use honey internally. However, I don't use or recommend that people substitute honey for maple syrup for the Master Cleanse. The maple syrup provides many alkaline minerals, including sodium, potassium, calcium, and magnesium, necessary to neutralize acidic toxins. I was once contacted by a man in India who couldn't find maple syrup, so he used honey. After the cleanse, he said his teeth became loose.

The USDA Nutrient Database says there is 14 times more calcium, 10 times more magnesium and 4 times more potassium in maple syrup compared to the same amount of honey. Don't use honey for the Master Cleanse.

If you cannot find maple syrup, use fresh sugar cane juice. Fresh sugar cane juice (notice, that is not cane syrup) is better than maple syrup and sorghum is worse than maple syrup. Diabetics should use molasses at first, then switch to maple syrup.

Person No. 69
What is the purpose of the maple syrup? Is it for energy?

Peter
Yes, plus the maple syrup provides many minerals, including sodium, potassium, calcium, magnesium, and others. It also provides Vitamins A, B1, B2, B6, C and Pantothenic Acid (B5).

Hunger vs. Cravings

Person No. 14
I am now on Day 7. To be honest the first three days were the best in terms of not being hungry. It has steadily gotten worse. Yesterday and today I am starving. Is this another detox sign? I thought hunger subsided. I am not craving anything. It's just a gnawing hunger and my stomach is constantly rumbling—even after the lemonade. Anyone else like this?

Person No. 70
I was in the same boat. The first time I did the cleanse I only lasted until Day 9 and was so hungry I couldn't stand it. I did everything the way I should have too. This time I tried to add more water. Drink a lemonade, drink a water. By Day 6, I was just getting hungrier and more miserable. So, I quit. Wish I could do it to Day 10, but for some reason I can't handle it. I had the same problem when I did a juice fast.

Peter

Frequently, people confused hunger with cravings. The way to distinguish between hunger and cravings is to ask yourself if you are interested in eating an apple, some carrots or a fresh green salad. If you are interested in those, you are hungry. If they are not appealing, but you are interested in ribs, French fries, a hamburger, etc., you are experiencing cravings. As cravings are a detox symptom, they will reduce or disappear with your next morning's eliminations if you are doing the Master Cleanse as written.

True hunger occurs in only about one quarter of the people doing the Master Cleanse. The rest feel no hunger at all no matter how long they cleanse. This is similar to people who do water fasts. Hunger disappears after Day 2 and doesn't reappear until the fast is complete. (This was one of my findings from a survey or 141 people who had done the Master Cleanse at one time or another.) It is possible these hungry people simply didn't drink enough lemonade or water. I have read that a single glass of water will turn off hunger in more than 90 percent of people on diets. Two people who experienced hunger, not cravings, that I talked to personally both had taken diet pills for some years. So it might have been due to detoxification of the diet pills. So I now know of four possibilities for hunger: 1) The person is not drinking another glass of lemonade or water, 2) The person is eating or drinking something in addition to the lemonade, salt water, or tea and that is creating or perpetuating the hunger; 3) The person is perceiving cravings as hunger; or 4) The person has a history of diet pills.

Hypoglycemia/Low Blood Sugar

People with hypoglycemia, or low blood sugar, are sometimes concerned because they have been told they have to eat every few hours. This is not a problem on the Master Cleanse provided you drink enough lemonade drinks to keep your blood sugar up in the first few days. After that, fasting (and the Master Cleanse is a juice fast) is known to normalize blood sugar so it will not be a problem later on the cleanse.

Infertility and the Cleanse

There are numerous mentions of infertility being handled by fasting. One for example is explained in the chapter, "Sterility In Women," in *Fasting Can Save Your Life* by Herbert M. Shelton. Shelton, a doctor of naturopathy (they teach how to use diet, exercise, lifestyle changes and natural therapies to enhance the body's ability to heal itself), fasted between 35,000 patients to health, including Joel Fuhrman, M.D., author of *Eat to Live*, who was inspired to become a doctor by this experience. Shelton tells of many cases where women, previously infertile and unable to conceive, conceived and delivered healthy children within a few weeks or months of fasting. I am aware of two women who were unable to conceive who did so within a few months of completing the Master Cleanse.

Interrupting the Cleanse

Peter
People have asked if they could "break" the cleanse with orange juice and/or grapefruit juice for a few days and then get back on it without losing the weight loss and cleansing benefits. I do not recommend it. Just orange juice or grapefruit juice might be okay for one day, but it will not sustain you for many days in a row.

Intestinal/Abdominal Cramps

Peter
Due to less waste in the intestines, you can sometimes feel intestinal contractions. Occasionally, they are uncomfortable. This can be handled by drinking more lemonade or water to give the intestines something to push. This generally handles it within a few minutes. Long term, use an herbal tea that is a combination of herbs rather than pure senna leaf or only drink half of the cup of laxative tea.

January Cleanse

Peter
[In the middle of December 2003, my wife and I decided to promote a Master Cleanse in January 2004 to help people recover from the excesses of the holidays. I had set a goal of 100 people doing the cleanse that month. We actually had 100 people on the bulletin board cleansing and I knew of ten more that did not have a connection to the Internet. So, they could not post to the bulletin board.

Person No. 10
I've done this many times and love it. My experience has always been about the same—one or two days of discomfort, headaches and hunger.

The next few days are great and then Days 8 onward are fantastic. It is more than about food. It becomes about how blessed I am in all areas of my life. God Bless and Happy New Year!

Person No. 37
I am so happy to see several people with the same idea as I have. I am starting the Master Cleanse today and plan on doing it quarterly. It's the best thing for my body. I felt great after my first cleanse.

Person No. 38
I am going to start my first time Master Cleanse on Monday, the 5th of January. My husband says he's going to do it with me. I hope so since he's seen what a difference a recent raw food/juice cleanse did for me at an institute in San Diego, where a raw foods lifestyle was introduced to me. I love the way it made me feel and want to incorporate more of it into our lives. I was happy to find your website. Thank you.

Person No. 39
I am on Day 9. One more day left, then orange juice and soup! I've had these wonderful things happen to me while on the cleanse:

1. I lost 10 lbs.

2. I no longer have to get surgery on knee as the toxin buildup is gone!

3. My blemishes cleared up and my overall skin is soft and smooth.

4. I had a mental, physical, and spiritual awakening!

This worked GREAT for me! I'm looking forward to organic food!

Person No. 40
I'm on my fourth day, I feel great and have really begun to notice a change in my sensory conditions, i.e. smell, taste, hearing, etc. WOW!

Person No. 7
I'm on Day 6 and feel very relaxed and in touch with my surroundings. This is my second attempt to do the Master Cleanse. The first time I was doing shift work and found it too difficult to go through the whole ten days. After speaking to many friends and reading all your comments, I came to the conclusion this is something I must experience. Drinking the lemonade is great. I love lemons, maple syrup and spicy foods. My cravings have finally disappeared and I am anxious to see what changes my body will go through in the next few days. Good health to all.

Person No. 41

I just want to let you know that I will be starting the cleanse tomorrow—January 16. This bulletin board has already been a real encouragement to me in my quest for healthy eating. I would like to become a raw vegan this year and this fast seems like the best way to start. I've read quite a bit about fasting and this seems to put a lot of the concepts together in a very workable method, so I guess I'll find out. I'm working on my husband and others to try to get them to participate in this fast also. We'll see if I can bump the number up. I'll be checking back in. Thanks.

Person No. 24

I am having a hard time drinking enough lemonade. I only drank four cups yesterday and only two so far today and it's already 4:00 p.m. Any thoughts? I look forward to more communing with The Master Cleansers! Love and light.

Person No. 11

What I have done to make sure I drink at least six glasses is I have left four lemons on my kitchen counter (four small lemons are enough for six glasses of lemonade). If they are gone by the end of the day, I know I have done okay. Good luck. I am on Day 5 and feeling great!

Person No. 24

Thank you so much for responding! I was feeling at a loss when I looked up to see if anyone had responded to me. Support helps a lot! Great to hear Day 5 is good. I think I will go take a shower and maybe a walk. If I can just make it through tonight, I will deal with tomorrow when it comes.

Peter

The first two or three days are always the worst because the toxins from the most recent waste are right there to be eliminated and when the toxins are eliminated, the body craves whatever is in the toxins: hamburgers, cheese, etc. So, it's usually easy to do the rest of the cleanse.

Person No. 17

I decided to get in on the January cleanse. This has been my first-ever day on my first-ever cleanse. It went okay, except I am already bored of the lemonade. Oh well, one day at a time. Gonna drink my lax tea and hit the sack. Thanks for the bulletin board. It is very helpful.

Peter

Boredom is a detox symptom. When you get past the first two or three days, you'll feel wonderful. That's your natural state. Boredom is the result of toxins in your body.

Person No. 12

Count me in your January "100." I started January 17, 2004. A friend of mine introduced it to me and she's a couple days ahead of me. We are a support system. My husband won't do it, but he is being very supportive. I love this site and I will continue to post questions and comments. I am on Day 3, slightly hungry, but in complete control so far. Reading the board, I see it gets better with time. Thank goodness!

Person No. 32

Hi Peter,

I met you at the raw food meeting in Clearwater this month and was planning on a three-day water fast, but after hearing you speak, I decided to do the Master Cleanse with a friend who was also at the meeting. You can count us in as part of the 100. We are on Day 6.

Prior to starting the cleanse, I ate just fruits and vegetables for three days in an attempt to cleanse a bit so that I wouldn't have bad toxic symptoms from all that sugar I ate at during the holidays. I was feeling headachy the night before the cleanse, and the entire first day. It was pretty bad and I really laughed at myself when I contemplated taking aspirin. The next morning, the headache traveled to the other side of my head, but by mid-morning it was gone. What a relief!

My aunt visited for the first five days of my fast, and left this morning. It was hard feeding her and my children—not seeing the food, but smelling it. I find that it makes me irritable to smell the food and not eat it. I suppose that's common. I'm hanging in there. Thanks for being here!

Peter

A pure raw vegetable and fruit diet also detoxifies. If you don't handle the other side of the program (elimination), you can end up with detox symptoms like headaches, irritability, boredom, cravings, etc. It's actually easier just to do the cleanse.

As far as it being difficult to feed others, that usually disappears around Day 8. A good friend, after Day 7, helped a friend of his, a chef, prepare grilled pork tenderloins for dinner and my friend on the cleanse wasn't bothered at all!

Thanks for posting on this bulletin board. It helps others to know how many are doing this. For example, this board was started on Dec. 29, 2003 and already (Jan. 21, 2004) over 1100 (not a typographic error) people have read this topic!

Person No. 42
I am on Day 3 of my cleanse. I just found this site, it has already answered some of the things I was wondering about.

Person No. 32
Today is Day 8 and I'm happy to report that making dinner for my kids tonight didn't bother me at all. I am also extremely pleased to say that there has been a shift in my thinking today—about lots of things. I am much more serene and peaceful. The spiritual side of the fast is emerging and it feels wonderful! Thanks again for this board.

Person No. 43
Hello, I just completed my first day of the cleanse and intend to go more than ten days if possible. I have this strange ambition to do a forty-day cleanse. Odd, huh?

Peter
It's not a strange thought at all. I've often wondered about doing a forty-day cleanse myself. The benefits after Day 8 for me have all been spiritual: more clarity of purpose; the ability to face stress without turning to food as a comfortable avoidance mechanism; the ability to smell wonderful smells (ribs for me) without the compulsion to eat it—much like you wouldn't eat a bar of soap or a scratch n' sniff just because it smelled good. Many native cultures use fasts as a spiritual tool.

Person No. 33
My husband and I have joined the January cleanse. We are on Day 9. It is the first time for us both. I have fasted many times but was unable to do the lemonade fast before because I felt sick each time I tried. I was happy to find your website to hear about your challenge and am happy to report this time has been a success.

It has been a great challenge. The first three days found us in the bathroom often. My husband is about to stop and will be undertaking a raw food diet. I have decided to stay a few more days. I have been monitoring my detox and I believe I have some more time to go. I have a slight headache this morning. A few days ago I had drainage from my eyes and there appears to be a rash on my face. So I think I will continue until the rash goes away and my face clears up. Thanks for the challenge.

Peter
Good for you!

A detox day (rash, drainage, etc.) is not a day to stop. You'll be happy afterward.

Person No. 44
I am on Day 6 and I feel great. I am amazed that I did this. I am a construction worker and a bathroom is not always available so I must end my cleanse before I go back to work in three days. Today I will have orange juice. I already made the vegetable soup for tomorrow. I wish I could stay on this cleanse for more days as I feel better each day. I can breathe better and the dry skin on my hands has disappeared. I am shocked at what still leaves my body as I have not had food for six days. Gross!

Peter
Many people are in the same situation. See the "Salt water flush" topic for a quote about using herbal laxative tea morning and evening rather than drinking the salt water. Then you could stay on the cleanse longer. The spiritual and mental clarity starts for me around Day 8.

Laxative Tea

Person No. 12
For Your Information: I am on Day 7. I was using a laxative tea that came in a cleanse pack that I purchased before this cleanse (parasite cleanse). I did not get nearly the great results I did when I switched to Smooth Move. It was about $3.49 at my nearest health food store. When I compared both teas Smooth Move had more senna in it than the other tea I was using. I suggest Smooth Move. To each his own—just make sure the tea has enough senna.

Person No. 3
This is my first time and I am on Day 2. I really haven't seen or felt any different, although I can barely get half of the salt water flush down. I have a question about the tea. Can I use any laxative tea or does it have to be a specific one? Thanks. This board has been very helpful.

Peter
No special one is recommended by Burroughs. I recommend a tea with about 50 percent senna leaf. You can find them at your local health food store.

Drink it only the last thing at night just before you go to sleep. It should take six to twelve hours before it causes eliminations. Sometimes it is faster. That way your eliminations will be right when you wake up in the morning instead of in the middle of the night.

Person No. 7
Cascara Sagrada is a beneficial herb (it's actually bark) that I have used and found it to be milder than senna. I took it in capsule form. I don't think it should effect the cleanse. Just take lots of water along with it.

Peter
Senna can be too powerful when there is not much in the colon to expel. Switch to a senna blend (50 percent senna and 50 percent other herbs) or make only half a cup of senna and then dilute it with mint tea or water. Cascara Sagrada is not a good solution as it is too bitter to make into a tea and taking it in capsules (the usual method) requires digestion and slows the cleanse.

Person No. 45
I'm planning to start the cleanse on Saturday, but I have a concern regarding the SWF and laxative tea: after doing the flush and taking the tea for as long as I do the cleanse, is there a danger that my bowel will have become dependent on these, leading to problems after the cleanse?

Peter
I have never heard of anyone who has become dependent on either the salt water flush or the laxative tea from doing the Master Cleanse. I imagine it could happen, but then there are people who cannot live without a candy bar every meal, too.

Lemonade, Amount to Drink

Person No. 46
This is my second day. When I mix up a pitcher of the lemonade, can I just pour myself a glass whenever I want, as long as I drink up to twelve glasses a day? Thank you! It's only my second day, but I feel such a great change already.

Peter

When you mix up a pitcher of the lemonade, you can drink the lemonade whenever you want. I would wait at least a half hour to one hour after the salt water. Finish drinking it at least two hours before going to sleep. Then you don't have to wake up to use the bathroom. Drink the laxative tea just before you go to sleep. These are not Master Cleanse instructions, just my suggestions.

Lemonade, Premixing

Person No. 47

Do any of you premix a jug of lemonade to take to work with you, or is this a definite no-no?

Person No. 8

I don't know if it is a no-no or not but I make up a gallon at a time. Then I put it all in eleven-ounce bottles I have so I can just grab a couple of bottles and go out the door. Today I went shopping and took two bottles of juice and two of water and I was gone for six hours. I was hungry when I got home but just made and drank some more. Good luck.

Peter

**Let's face it. You have to premix enough to last through the day if you are going to go to work outside your house. However, I have heard of people squeezing lemons and mixing the maple syrup as a "premix" that they then add to water over the next two or more days. (Never use commercial bottled juice! It is pasteurized and old = no enzymes.) If you have read anything about the wheatgrass diet, the Hippocrates diet, the raw food diet, the Gerson anti-degenerative disease regimen, juicing for health or the Optimum Health Institute, you know that enzymes diminish over time, even in as little time as a few hours. You cannot get away from having to make enough to get through the day, but making more than one day's supply (even a day and an evening) will diminish your benefits. Also, if you do make a premix daily, do not add the cayenne until you are ready to drink. Cayenne will get hotter as it sits in liquid.

Person No. 34

I like to have my juice really fresh to get the full benefit of the enzymes in the lemons. However, I work an eight-hour day. So, what I do is make up a batch for just work. I usually drink three to four servings in that time. I do the lemon, maple syrup and water but not the cayenne pepper yet. I then pour myself one serving in a portable cup and add the pepper to just the one glass. Otherwise, the pepper gets too hot. When I pour myself a new glass at work, I add the pepper to that glass. Then when I come home at the end of the day, I just make one serving at a time.

Lemons, Buying in Quantity

Person No. 9

I'm starting the cleanse this weekend and after reading the topics, it looks like it's going to take around six or seven lemons a day. What is the shelf-life of lemons for the purpose of the cleanse? (I'm not sure if the beneficial properties break down while they are in the fridge.)

Also, I don't see too many people mentioning limes. Is there a big difference? Can you alternate just to shake things up a bit? Thanks!

Peter

A large lemon will yield two ounces of juice. So, for six drinks a day, you will need three large lemons per day or thirty for ten days. If you buy organic lemons, only get enough for five days as that is the longest they last in the refrigerator. Limes are great for a change of pace. They are smaller and you will need about twice as many of them to make a drink. Burroughs says you can use either lemons or limes. I prefer the taste of lemons for the long run, but occasional drinks with lime are kind of fun.

Lemons, Juicing

Person No. 43

I'm on Day 5 and eating just seems so trivial at this point. I feel great and my energy is off the charts. I found a way of satisfying that need for "something solid." When I make my lemonade, instead of squeezing the lemon, I just blend it in a blender (without the peel). The pulp gives me the sensation that I'm eating something whole. Come to think of it, is that okay? I figured it would be, seeing as how some people blend the pulp and peel into the drink.

Peter

Yes, blending some of the skin (organic lemons only) and pulp can enhance the lemon's effectiveness. Also, if there is any internal bleeding, this will enhance the lemon's ability to reduce bleeding and prevent clotting internally. (It doesn't, however, interfere with normal menstrual periods.) You must peel the rind on non-organic ones. Then put the whole thing through the juicer.

Person No. 14

Maybe a stupid question. Does it make any difference to the effectiveness of the lemons how you squeeze them? I have been using a Champion juicer and getting quite a bit of juice that way, but last night I couldn't be bothered to do it that way and used a plain old lemon squeezer. The juice tasted different. Anyone know if there's a best way or if it makes no difference?

Peter

I have done it two ways: using an expensive juicer with whole organic lemons and with just squeezing the lemons. The taste is quite different, but I got the same results both ways.

Person No. 21

This bulletin board is a wonderful source for information and support. I've really enjoyed reading the posts. I have a question. Is it ok to use "bottled" lemon juice instead of fresh organic lemons? I've been using fresh lemons, but I'm going through them fast and where I live lemons are kind of expensive. Also, are there inexpensive places to buy the organic maple syrup and lemons?

Peter

Bottled juice is a no-no as the vitamins and enzymes that do the good work are destroyed by time, sunlight and cooking (pasteurizing). Even if you find non-pasteurized "raw" or frozen lemon juice, after several hours most of the enzymes are destroyed by time.

Concerning the high prices of organic ingredients for the cleanse, realize you are not buying any other food. Although organic is not required, it is well worth it. When you finish the cleanse, you will discover that you don't eat as much quantity any more, so rather than eat foods that have had all their enzymes and vitamins removed and then had preservatives and pesticides added, why not spend the same money for fewer high-quality (organic) foods with real nutrition?

One of the things I have learned from my research into nutrition and healing is that proper nutrition equals a pleasant, serene attitude toward life. The spiritual side starts to show through.

Person No. 48
Peter, I read your article in *Natural Awakenings* magazine and am so
excited to start the cleanse! Must you use organic lemons or limes or
can you just not use the rinds? Thanks so much.

Peter
It is not required to use organic lemons or limes. If you are only
squeezing them and not putting them through a juicer, you needn't
peel the rind on non-organic ones. That is only if you are going to put
the whole thing through the juicer.

Length of Cleanses and Time Between Them

Person No. 49
How often should one do the cleanse? Is there a difference between a
five-day and a twenty-day fast?

Peter
Not only does the Master Cleanse make the body healthier, it also
temporarily gives peace of mind and a sense of peaceful energy. My
first cleanse was for twenty days. I have also done this cleanse for two
and three days. Burroughs says to do the cleanse for a minimum of ten
days. He doesn't say why, but here are my thoughts. Days 2 and 3 are
generally the worst because the body hasn't yet switched to burning fat
(scientifically called going into ketosis). Day 7 is the first time old waste
is eliminated, so this is usually a day with noticeable detox symptoms.
The real gains start after Day 7.

So, doing it for three days or less is feeling unpleasant with no actual
old waste eliminated. At least eliminate some of the old waste and
give yourself a few days of really enjoying the feeling of energy and
happiness. That is ten days.

A twenty-day cleanse produced, for me and many others, temporary
spiritual gains beyond just health. This cleanse is like pressing reset for
the body. It puts everything back to normal.

Person No. 50
Peter, what is a major detox day? What are your symptoms? Thanks.

Peter
A major detox day is one where you have noticeable symptoms. [See
the topic "Detox Symptoms—the Good, the Bad and the Ugly" for
more info.]

Person No. 16
Is there anything unhealthy about doing the cleanse and eating raw food on alternate days? It would keep my body clean and I would continue losing weight.

Peter
Burroughs recommends drinking the Master Cleanse lemonade in the morning as a health regimen even after the cleanse. He also recommends a predominantly raw fruit, vegetable, seed, nut and berry diet.

Alternating one day each of a raw vegan diet and the Master Cleanse doesn't seem like a good idea to me. On the Master Cleanse, there is a detox day on about the seventh day. So staying on it for ten days makes a lot of sense to maximize the detoxifying effect.

As for the raw vegan diet, raw food author and lecturer, Victoria Boutenko, says it takes a week before the red blood cells recover from eating cooked food. In one of her recent lectures in Clearwater, Florida, she showed slides of red blood cells that were spherical and surrounded on all sides by plasma and then those taken one half hour after eating cooked food. In the latter slides, the red blood cells were all jammed together and no longer spherical. She said it takes a week for the red blood cells to return to their natural healthy shape. The maple syrup in the Master Cleanse is not considered a raw food.

So, although I have found both of these health regimens to be valuable, combining them every other day would seem to defeat the purpose of each. I recommend you do the Master Cleanse when you want, and otherwise eat the raw vegan diet or have the Master Cleanse lemonade in the morning.

Madal Bal Syrup/Neera Cleanse

Peter
Here is what I know about Madal Bal syrup and the Neera Super Cleanse. In 2004, I recall they advertised Madal Bal syrup as a refinement by Stanley Burroughs himself and it was still called the Master Cleanse. Now it is called the Neera Super Cleanse and the story is that others in Europe researched a better syrup. The location of Europe is important. There is no maple syrup produced in Europe. So, the importing of maple syrup from the US or Canada would be very expensive. This may account for the use of an alternative in Europe. Furthermore, they claim that it includes Grade C maple syrup which is a grade no longer used by the US Dept. of Agriculture, which regulates the US grades, and Canada uses a numbered system.

Regardless of the above facts, it is much more expensive than maple syrup in the US and it is a questionable replacement. In countries where freshly extracted sugar cane juice is available, Burroughs says that is ideal. I personally stick with organic Grade B maple syrup, although I would love to try the freshly extracted sugar cane juice version if I could find it.

Maple Syrup, Loving It a Little Too Much

Person No. 15
I've been measuring out my lemonades exactly (on Day 3 now) and am finding myself leaving a little extra maple syrup left over in the measuring spoon after I pour so that I can lick it up. Is this totally wrong, since I'm not supposed to be giving into cravings? Or is it alright since I was just going to consume that little bit anyway? Plus, I'm only using a tablespoon and a half versus two in each lemonade, and drinking only six to seven lemonades daily, because I know I have such a sweet tooth. Okay, I'm not alone here folks, right? Who else is loving the pure sugary organic goodness of their maple syrup as much as I?

Person No. 13
Once or twice a day I will eat a tablespoon of the maple syrup by itself. I don't see how this can be wrong, other than as extra calories if you are overweight, but I am losing weight anyway since I am still taking in less calories by far than I normally would. I don't think this would hurt anything at all. All the maple syrup is doing is providing you with nutrients anyway.

Person No. 15
Yeah, I thought so. Thanks. I have had the desire to just eat a tablespoon by itself once or twice.

Person No. 6
I'm on Day 9 and I found quite a few little things that I enjoy and consider treats during the cleanse. I feel so guilty posting this, but such is life. I like to do a teaspoon of pure maple syrup every now and then. The other day I did a couple of teaspoons of molasses, but that was too good. So I put the molasses away until after the cleanse. Did I cheat? No, I just made it fun for me. Please do not follow these terrible, disgusting little nuances because indeed they are habit forming. Good luck to all!

Person No. 15

Okay, we all must agree that it's not wrong and continue to find ways to enjoy ourselves during the cleanse. What else do we have?

Peter

I didn't say anything when you talked about sneaking a teaspoon here or there as it didn't sound like you were establishing new rules for the cleanse. However, when you said, "We all must agree that it's not wrong and continue to find ways to enjoy ourselves during the cleanse," I thought I had better speak up. You were probably just having fun and it was not your intention to change the rules, but we do not know how many other people will read this topic and change the actual directions. I would like to avoid that.

I don't think it's the end of the world or going to destroy all the benefits of the cleanse to have a little extra maple syrup once or twice on the entire cleanse. However, I would like to make it clear that the Master Cleanse as written by Stanley Burroughs does not include any extra maple syrup.

I am sorry if I sound like a strict school teacher, but I have already seen how changes in the successful directions sneak in with misconceptions and wanted to be sure that others get the benefits they seek.

As to having a craving for additional maple syrup, try increasing the amount in the drink to the full two tablespoons rather than eating the maple syrup separately. This will keep your blood sugar level more constant and reduce your craving for an extra teaspoon of maple syrup now and then.

Maple Syrup Substitute

Person No. 31

I have been drinking mint herbal tea. It is hard to drink without some kind of sweetener so I add Equal. Is there anything wrong with this?

Peter

**For goodness sake, don't use any artificial sweeteners in your tea while on the Master Cleanse. Even after the cleanse, I would recommend dropping them. There are numerous studies on their ill effects.

I've heard Aspartame has been linked to some neurological degenerative diseases and may have something to do with fibromyalgia as well. As far as the cleanse is concerned, other than lemonade, salt water in the morning and laxative tea, plain mint tea is the only other thing mentioned by Stanley Burroughs in *The Master Cleanser*. I don't want to spoil your tea drinking, but while on the cleanse, you'll see more benefits if you stick to the cleanse as written.

Person No. 70
Hi all, great site. Can someone suggest a replacement for the maple syrup prescribed for the fast? I live in a smallish city in South Africa and absolutely cannot find maple syrup here at all. I'm afraid I've never seen any raw sugar cane stalks for sale anywhere. What do you think of using some other sweet juice as a last resort? I'm sure maple syrup would be best, but I guess we all have to do what we can. Many thanks.

Peter
**If you cannot find maple syrup, freshly extracted sugar cane juice makes the ideal lemonade drink. See the "Quick Start" section for the recipe. A less-than-optimum substitute is sorghum. Use two tablespoons, the same amount as maple syrup. Agave nector should not be used because it has more fructose than high fructose corn syrup.

Maple Syrup, Unable to Handle the Taste of

Person No. 36
My wife started this with me and very quickly could not handle the taste of the maple syrup. She said if she had another glass with that aftertaste she would vomit. Is there an alternative she could use?

Peter
The only other thing Burroughs talks about is cane juice (that's not cane syrup).

Person No. 13
Make sure she is using organic grade B maple syrup as well, because the taste difference is just astounding between this and regular maple syrup. I had never tried organic grade B before and was amazed at the taste. My mother didn't want to try it either because she hates maple syrup, but when she did she said, "Wow! That is really good." I figure you're probably using the right thing, but just make sure because the taste difference is huge.

Person No. 43
Yeah, Person No.13 makes a great point here. Conventional methods for producing maple syrup include formaldehyde. This drastically

reduces the taste and quality of maple syrup. I would suggest you make sure you have organic grade B maple syrup before you go out and buy cane juice.

Master Cleanse Beginner

Person No. 53

I like this forum because I can get in touch with others who are vegetarians, vegans, or raw foodists to decide what might be best for me.

I just started the cleanse yesterday and am very excited to see what happens. I have not read the book yet but plan to get it today. I was told about this cleanse by an acupuncturist. He told me I could have mint tea, is this true? Also, I didn't know I was supposed to start the cleanse with the salt water flush and I bought the wrong sea salt. It was iodized. So, I will get the right kind. I am so nervous doing this as I don't know the benefits, side effects, or even some of the smaller questions like, can I brush my teeth with toothpaste. I'm assuming not, so I haven't.

I have always been a healthy eater. However, for the last five months I was very bad and gained fifteen pounds. I am 5'2" and weigh 130. Will I lose healthy weight or muscle with the cleanse? Also, what do you think about the Blood Type Diet? I am a type B and have always eaten meat and dairy to keep down my weight. I've tried to be a vegetarian before and I gained weight. What do you suggest? I'm so sorry for all the questions. Your site is what has helped me so far and I really want to live healthily and inspire others with accurate information.

I couldn't do the salt water flush (SWF). It came back out. So, I bought Smooth Move (a laxative tea with senna and other herbs). Is this okay? My eliminations are mostly fluid. Is this normal? I don't know how I will be able to do the SWF as it makes me gag. Is there any other way? I have will power. However, once I drink it, it comes right back out! I really feel great already in three days. My skin is clearing up and I have a lot of energy! Hope to hear from you soon.

Peter

I'd recommend brushing your teeth with water only or bar soap and water and using the mint tea to freshen your mouth as quoted above.

Concerning losing healthy weight on the cleanse, Burroughs says the only thing you will lose is waste, not healthy tissue.

My personal opinion concerning eating protein and meat to keep weight off is that you are then eating too many acidic foods and throwing the body into an unhealthy situation. Burroughs promotes a raw fruit, nut and vegetable diet. So did Norman Walker, a naturopath who taught juicing and raw fruit and vegetable diets. He was active as a healer to the age of 100!

The salt water flush does indeed cause several eliminations within an hour or two (or longer for some people). The waste that is contained in the colon is impacted in layers and takes quite a while to detoxify and eliminate. Even though you are only seeing liquid (clear or yellow) for several days, you will pass some solid or semi-solid matter.

When I did a twenty-day Master Cleanse, I only passed solid waste on two or three days, but one of those was the seventeenth day. The "stuff" does indeed come off in layers and there's a lot there if you haven't done cleanses regularly for most of your life.

Is there another way besides the salt water flush? Yes. You can drink the laxative tea morning and night.

By the way, it is much easier to drink the salt water if you are using non-iodized sea salt rather than regular salt. My wife recommends using a straw if you want to avoid the super salty gag response. I've never needed to do that. So, I can't say if it works.

A senna blend tea such as Get Regular is perfect, although all Burroughs says is "herbal laxative tea."

That's great about your skin clearing up. The skin is one of the organs in the elimination system and in fact is the largest organ of the body. That it is clearing up means it is no longer overloaded with more toxic waste than it can handle.

Person No. 54
I have been using about three tablespoons of lemon juice with each glass for my own taste preference. I just read that you shouldn't alter the two tablespoons. Have I screwed up?

Peter
I doubt the extra lemon juice will ruin the cleanse. Whether it will yield the same excellent results is something I do not know. That is why I recommend following the Master Cleanse exactly as written. It works very well routinely.

If you want your lemonade less sweet, reduce the maple syrup. That is covered in the book.

Master Cleanse Book, Pass It Along

Person No. 55

Hi, all! I am brand spanking new. Heard about the Master Cleanse for the first time today. I am so excited to try this. I haven't gotten the book yet. I hope to get it tomorrow. I just have some quick questions. Can I have any herbal tea? Can I have chicken broth? Can I have V8 splash?

My friend did this with huge success. She wrote out an example day for me to follow:

Wake up: two glasses lemonade; Breakfast: herbal tea, lemonade; Snack: herbal tea, lemonade; Lunch: chicken broth; Snack: herbal tea, lemonade; Dinner: fresh fruit juice, lemonade; Snack: herbal tea, lemonade. So that's the day she gave me.

Is this ok? I'm afraid I won't have time to get the book tomorrow. I have a five-year-old and a six-month-old. I am not breast feeding and also work part-time in the evenings. I just don't want to start out doing the wrong thing.

This board is awesome and I am so excited I found it! If any of you could help me out, that would be so great. Thanks guys.

Peter

You will be surprised when you read the book because there is no chicken broth or fruit juice and your friend didn't mention the salt water flush in the morning.

I strongly recommend everyone who wants to do the Master Cleanse read the book. Verbal directions are like playing telephone, where you whisper something to someone who whispers what they heard to someone else, etc. down the line for five or ten people. The message is never the same.

I want you to get the best possible results. That will come by doing exactly what Stanley Burroughs developed. If you do not know what that is, you cannot be sure you are going to get the results you want.

Person No. 71

I read about this in a magazine and was intrigued. I looked it up on the web and started. I have never done a MC before. I have done a juice fast and detoxed other ways. I am excited about this, but I have two questions.

1. I did not read the book when beginning. The article I read said it was okay to have one twelve-ounce drink of organic fresh juice and one twelve-ounce bowl of fresh organic veggie broth. Is this okay or should I stop?

2. I have done the salt water internal bath. It worked well. That was a first. How many times should I do this? I am assuming from what I have read, every day?

Peter

1. Yes, you should stop drinking the fresh juice and veggie broth. The Master Cleanse as developed and written by Stanley Burroughs includes nothing but salt water in the a.m., six to twelve glasses daily of the lemon- or limeade, one cup of herbal laxative tea at night (and, optionally, one more in the morning), mint tea occasionally, and blackstrap molasses for diabetics during the cleanse. He does talk about slowly drinking several eight ounce glasses of fresh orange juice as desired throughout the day *after* completing the cleanse to break it. (Personally, I find the orange juice too heavy after the cleanse and prefer grapefruit juice.) He recommends a veggie broth soup as the evening meal on the second day after the cleanse. He gives a recipe for the soup in *The Master Cleanser* on page 26.

2. Yes, the salt water flush is done each morning of the cleanse. The worksheet on **www.TheMasterCleanse.com** (and earlier in this book) gives you the items and the times to use them.

You should also be drinking the herbal laxative tea each evening as you'll see on the worksheet. By the way, the worksheet is not meant to replace the book. The book has lots of other valuable information.

Person No. 16

I am in high school. I get up at 5:00 in the morning and leave the house at 6:10, I can't do the salt in the morning because I don't think I will have enough time to let it work. Can I do the salt flush when I come home, usually 3:30 p.m., but some days at 5:30? I know you said not to flush so that the lemonade and pepper can work overnight, but I don't have any of the pepper! Don't you think the flush will work and be done at 5:00? I also wanted to know if sarsaparilla tea is good enough.

Peter

That is great that you are taking such good care of your body at your age. If you cannot do the flush, drink the herb laxative tea night and morning like the book says.

You must go to the store and buy some cayenne pepper. It is sold as red pepper. It helps to dissolve the mucus and build the blood. It also opens the blood vessels to increase the flow of nutrients to the body's cells. It's not the Master Cleanse without it. It is quite inexpensive.

Sarsaparilla tea is not a laxative. Herbal references say that sarsaparilla is good for gout and rheumatism and is very similar to testosterone in the body, but it is not a laxative. Licorice root is a mild laxative. Senna is a stronger one. Go to the health food store and buy a combination tea with both of those in it.

Please buy the book and read it. It sounds like you're missing the mark with no salt water, no cayenne and drinking sarsaparilla tea. I want you to get all the benefits you can.

Please, when you care enough about others' health to tell them about the Master Cleanse, please care enough to see they read the book. Give it to them, send them to **www.TheMasterCleanse.com**, or send them to a store to buy it. From the above postings to the bulletin board, you can see the misinformation that gets passed on when the book is not used as the source of how to do the Master Cleanse.

Medication

Person No. 56

I take Wellbutrin for minimal depression. Should I still take it or discontinue it for the fast?

Peter

I'm not a medical doctor and even if I were, I don't have your complete medical history, chart and any diagnostic test results. So, I would not even dream of advising you as to whether you should discontinue your medicine. You should seek the advice of your licensed health care provider and use your own good judgment.

Here is some information that you may find useful to help make your decision.

1. The purpose of a cleanse is to remove toxins and old waste from the body. The body in most cases treats medical drugs as toxins from a

digestive standpoint. So, putting more in while trying to get toxins out doesn't make a lot of sense. Thus, you may consider eliminating any NON-PRESCRIBED medicines, such as allergy, diet or sleeping pills that were not prescribed by a licensed healthcare professional. If you are on a prescribed medication, especially such as that to avoid a heart attack, stroke or other fatal event, do NOT discontinue your medicine without consulting a licensed healthcare practitioner, or getting a second opinion. Remember, there are many kinds of licensed healthcare practitioners: chiropractors, naturopaths, acupuncturists, doctors of oriental medicine, nutritionists, etc. If you are on medication for high blood pressure, know that fasting has been scientifically shown to reduce blood pressure. So, you will very likely have to adjust your dosage. In the same way, those on blood thinners should know that cayenne pepper acts as a blood thinner, which may require adjusting dosages as well. Anyone on chemotherapy or anti-depressants should see those topics.

2. In some cases, the body stores some of the medicine it is taking in the fat cells. Max Gerson, M.D. (www.gerson.org), reported that a percentage of each dose of chemotherapy medicine is stored in the body and could be released during detoxification. I believe this is likely with strong psychiatric medicines also. I recommend people who have been on chemotherapy or strong psychiatric medicines within the last six months do a much gentler and slower detox. You can always come back to the Master Cleanse later after you have done a slower form of detox.

3. As far as doing the cleanse while being on the medication, in a January 2005 survey of 141 people who have done or were doing the Master Cleanse, only one person reported having any problems at all with her medication. And that lady only had a problem once, but went on and did the cleanse nine more times!

I'm sorry I can't give you a yes or no answer, but I hope this helps.

Person No. 72
Peter, I read your article in *Natural Awakenings*, researched the Master Cleanse on the web, and went to your website as mentioned in the article. Thanks for providing this website. It was a great blessing to me, a first time MCer. In fact, my mother, seventy-one years old, and my brother, forty-three years old, and sister, thirty years old, will be doing the MC for the first time starting in February.

My mother is on medication. She takes blood pressure and blood thinning medications. I told her to do the MC gradually, in small time allocations (this first time she is only doing a thirty-six-hour cleanse), then listen to her body and see how she feels. She has a doctor's appointment scheduled a day after she breaks her fast. Her goal is to be able to do a thirty-six-hour fast once a month for a while, then progress to a three-day fast, then a five-day fast, etc. until her health will allow her to complete the minimum ten-day fast in the future, perhaps next year this time.

Peter

The one person I know who had high blood pressure going into the cleanse noticeably reduced it on the cleanse and kept it lower (although not as low as while on the cleanse) with a raw vegetarian diet.

Have her run the concept of the cleanse lowering blood pressure by her doctor for coordination purposes to make sure she doesn't get a double whammy from the combined effects of the medication and the cleanse and faint when she stands up. Fasting is known to reduce high blood pressure. In fact, there is a scientific study done on 174 people with high blood pressure. After a ten-day water fast, everyone on medication was able to come off it. Be sure she stands or sits slowly. I think the idea of short cleanses until she's stable is a good idea.

**Be advised that the Master Cleanse will also thin the blood. So, if she is on blood-thinning medication, she will need to work with her licensed healthcare practitioner to adjust dosages. I spoke to a man recently who loved what the Master Cleanse did for him, but he was pulled off it twice by his doctor who had him on a blood thinner and his tests showed it was too thin each time on the Master Cleanse. That doctor refused to adjust his dosage. So, he found another doctor willing to adjust it while he was on the Master Cleanse.

Person No. 72

Thanks for your response. My mom is so excited. She will actually start the thirty-six-hour Master Cleanse Monday, Feb. 2, 2004. After that, depending on how she feels she may extend the cleanse a few more days. I will keep a close eye on her and cheer her on when she starts getting detox symptoms and will want to quit. She has been using medications for years. We will take it slow.

Regarding her blood pressure medication, the doctor has scheduled her every three months, the first appointment the first Friday in February, to monitor it in order to reduce the dose as required. I think the MC is the best thing that ever happened to her and me for that matter. I enlighten everyone that I come in contact with. Thanks again Peter. May God bless you and your entire family!

Person No. 54

I have been on a low dose of Zoloft for the past three years. I am continuing to take it. I'm on Day 5. Will it somehow interfere with the cleanse?

Peter

See my reply at the beginning of this topic to Person No. 56. In addition, I recommend the book *Potatoes, not Prozac* by Kathleen DesMaisons (available at **www.TheMasterCleanse.com**). It explains how a proper diet can address mental distress that is actually caused by the wrong diet.

Minerals

Person No. 49

I currently take all natural liquid magnesium chloride. I know that the maple syrup has some magnesium, but wanted to know if it would be okay to take the liquid magnesium (one-half teaspoon) with the drink. It is not a pill, therefore it would not need to be as digested as a pill would, correct?

Peter

The maple syrup, cayenne and lemon provide all the minerals needed for daily function and cleansing. The lemon also acts as a blood alkalizer. I recommend you follow the cleanse as written and abstain from any supplements until after the cleanse. *The Master Cleanser* by Stanley Burroughs says you do not need and should not take any supplements while on the cleanse.

Mucoid Plaque

[Mucoid plaque is a tough rubbery coating that forms from mucus and accumulated waste on the large intestine walls. There are numerous pictures of this on the Web.]

Person No. 13

I want to see this [referring to a picture on the web] come out of me, more than anything. How many people here have shed mucoid? I saw that one person did, on another topic. Should I expect to definitely see this happen if I stay on the fast for about twenty days? Or, do you think it comes out regardless on the cleanse, maybe just not all in one piece like that?

Person No. 12
Hey girl, I have not seen that yet and I am on Day 4. If that's what's inside me, I'll be happy when I see it come out! GOOD LAWD! That must be a scary sight!

Person No. 11
I am on Day 9 and I haven't seen that horror yet!

Person No. 13
Well, that usually comes from doing a typical colon cleanse with lots of supplements and colonics. But, I am hoping this cleanse will get rid of it just as well. Maybe it just doesn't take that form. Maybe it just comes out in smaller pieces instead of all at once, like I said. I hope so. Anyone else with feedback about this, please reply.

Peter
I've only heard of one person who described an elimination that could have been mucoid plaque and that person fit the description of someone who ate the SAD diet and had never done a cleanse, colonic, nor eaten a raw food diet.

Most times, the accumulated waste is just dissolved over several days by the lemon juice and cayenne, washed by the salt water, and broken up into small mucousy flakes by the increased intestinal action brought on by the herbal laxative tea. That's always been the case for me. Even after seventeen days of not eating, I've had mucousy flakes eliminated.

I think anyone wanting to see foot-long sections (or longer) of mucoid plaque needs to do a colon cleanse with psyllium and/or bentonite clay that mechanically pushes the waste out rather than the Master Cleanse, which dissolves it. Personally, I prefer the Master Cleanse.

Person No. 13
Well, I was hoping that it just got broken into pieces. I don't care how it comes out, just as long as it does. I would much rather have it come out gradually than have to sit on the toilet for hours and have it all come out in one big piece like it does with a traditional colon cleanse. I'm not patient enough for that.

Nothing Happening

Person No. 12

I am on Day 5. No solid bowel movement, no weight loss, no increase in energy. The only thing is that I'm not groggy in the morning and have weird dreams! That's it. I'm going to continue and not give up, but I am getting frustrated. My girlfriend lost nine pounds in the first four days. Ugh!

Peter

Well, let's look at all the points where this cleanse could go wrong and see if we can sort it out.

1. Are you putting two teaspoons of non-iodized sea salt in the salt water each morning and drinking it as fast as possible?

2. Are you mixing two tablespoons (one ounce) of *fresh squeezed*—not bottled—lemon juice into each ten-ounce drink or using these proportions for each batch and making no more than one day's worth at a time?

3. Are you putting in at least 1/10 teaspoon of cayenne pepper or less and gradually increasing the amount to taste with each drink?

4. Are you drinking one cup of laxative tea each morning as well as each evening to encourage more elimination?

5. Are you eating or drinking anything else but water and occasional mint tea?

6. Before this cleanse, did you have only one or two BMs per week? Being constipated before the cleanse might mean a little longer before you would see results.

7. Are you on any constipating medications? I am NOT suggesting you come off any prescribed medications. Just that they may alter the results of the cleanse. The only other thought I have for anyone not seeing results by Day 5 is that some people who have lived on the SAD diet (Standard American Diet) and are overweight may take a while before enough accumulated waste is loosened and eliminated to start seeing results. Go for the full ten days. That is what Burroughs says. Big changes usually come after Day 7.

Person No. 12

Peter, Thanks for the input. You helped me out a LOT. Ok here are my faults:

1) On Days 1-4 I had been using two tablespoons of salt, not teaspoons. I used two teaspoons today (Day 5) and it has not come out yet.

2) I am using an herbal tea only at night, NOT MORN—I will increase that to a morning cup.

3) I've always been a once a day bathroom girl, so I think it may take longer for me.

4) I am using a laxative herbal tea with senna, but not Smooth Move. The one I've been using contains other herbs as well as added vitamins (I think vitamin C). I will switch teas to Smooth Move and start taking one cup at night and in the morning.

I can say I am doing the drink correctly. I measure my lemonade drinks perfectly and I use organic lemons and maple syrup with plenty of cayenne. I usually drink six to ten glasses a day and about sixty-four to ninety-six ounces of water in between!

My only other concern—I use Crystal Springs Mountain bottled water from the store. Is this ok?

Peter

The bottled water is okay so long as it does not contain fluoride.

Person No. 16

I suggest Yellow Dock tea because it is just as effective as any senna blend and it is fast acting, painless and smooth, whereas senna can cause intestinal spasms.

If you're worried about taste though, don't use Yellow Dock because it tastes literally like the bark of a tree. But I kind of like that because I'm a very strict vegan/raw vegan and I like to taste pure nature. Good luck!!

For the first few days, I had no bowel movements. However, I just added a little more tea to my water and now I make a few. I am losing weight, too. I'm on the sixth day and I've lost nine pounds.

Since I'm writing a comment here, I might as well ask my question: I know that in the book Burroughs says that fatty tissue melts away and is eliminated, but another place in the book he says nothing but toxins and diseases are eliminated, so I just wanted to know if some of the weight I'm losing is actual.

Peter
Toxins are primarily stored in the fat. This is one of the reasons for so many overweight Americans. It is the result of their SAD diet. The preservatives, artificial colors and flavors and other non-real-food that they eat are treated by the body as toxins. What it cannot eliminate, it stores in fat cells. Lose the toxins...lose the fat!

Person No. 16
What about this quote on page thirteen, "As a reducing diet it is superior in every way to any other system because it dissolves and eliminates all types of fatty tissue. Fat melts away at the rate of about two pounds a day for most persons—and without any harmful side effects."

Peter
When you release the toxins with the cleanse or eating only a raw vegetarian diet, the fat is no longer needed as the toxins are gone and the body sheds the fat.

Person No. 17
I'm on the end of Day 4, but don't feel like I am gaining a lot more energy, losing any weight or having any real positive results. I know I am detoxing based on the last two days. I felt good the first two days and Day 3 was weird. I had mild tingling sensations in different body parts, a jaw ache, a mild sore throat, a groggy brain and food cravings. Today was just the worst, only because I wanted to eat sooooo bad. Everything looked good.

My BMs seem normal, getting some waste out each morning. I am doing everything (almost) as prescribed in the book, laxative tea at night, salt water flush in the morning, but here is my concern. I can barely manage to get down six cups of lemonade a day. (Some days it has been five and one-quarter). When I do finish a cup I notice a lot of the pepper seems to be left at the bottom and I do not drink the pepper-filled last ounce in the cup. Yuck!

In fact, I cheat a bit on the pepper because it tastes so bad and only put in 1/16 tsp. instead of the prescribed 1/10th. After all, who has a 1/10 measuring spoon? This has to be a bit of a guess for most doesn't it? (Don't advise the cayenne pills, I don't swallow pills well.)

Anyway, I wonder how just barely drinking the minimum affects the cleanse and is using just slightly less pepper a big deal? Does it stand to reason that if you are a small person it would be sufficient to drink less than if you weighed a 100 lbs. more? Just a hopeful thought.

If anyone has any comments on how they manage to get in seven or more cups I would love to hear.

Thanks for reading this lengthy message. Reading all of your messages has given me some encouragement at a time when I really need it.

Peter
Hi Person No.17, those are good questions.

If you don't drink the minimum, you won't detoxify as much or as fast. Lots of fluids help cleanse the kidneys and liver as well as the colon. One way to get down more lemonade is to drink only lemonade until you reach your minimum of six drinks. Drink your first glass about one-half to one hour after the salt water. Then drink a glass every hour. This will make you pee frequently. Every time you pee, drink another glass.

On the cayenne, it speeds everything up. It dilates blood vessels, breaks up the mucus and increases circulation and metabolism. You are quite correct: it is all estimation regarding measuring the cayenne. **Do not put so much in that you hate the taste of the lemonade and then can't drink it. However, do try to stretch your tolerance of it.

It is important to mix up the lemonade just before you drink it, so you get the cayenne. Not getting enough cayenne will definitely slow down your cleanse. I mix up the cayenne by making up four drinks at a time in a large plastic bottle and shaking the bottle every time just before I drink it.

The other thing to understand is that this is a ten-day process. Yes, some people get results more quickly than others, but do not judge your results by what happens after five, six or seven days.

Take a longer view. If you get enough lemonade and cayenne, you'll not be straining to try to make it to Day 6. You'll be cruising with the rest of us.

By the way, the minimum for smaller people is six drinks per day, not seven. Hope this helps.

Person No. 13

If all else fails, hold your nose and chug! I started doing this when I started drinking green veggie juice (kale, collard, cucumber, celery) which tastes awful, but is awesome for you. It also helps to think of what you're taking as medicine, because it is—just like when you were a child and would hold your nose for medicine. Think of it the same way and this doesn't taste nearly as bad as most of that stuff.

As far as the pepper goes, just mix it up really well, and chug, chug, chug, even if you have trouble doing this at first. Your breathing and throat will adjust so that you can.

Person No. 17

Peter and Person No.13, thank you both for your responses. Today was a better day. I quit drinking the lemonade in a cup and have switched to a bottle with a straw and that seems to help me drink it faster. I might try the nose-holding thing if I really want to chug. But the pepper burns my throat and makes me cough sometimes.

Well, finishing Day 5 makes me feel like I am over the hump. It can only get better from here, right? Thanks for the ideas and encouragement. I appreciate it.

Person No. 47

I'm on Day 5 of the MC. Have been doing it just as the book says—the salt water every morning, lemonade during the day, and Smooth Move tea at night. I have a few questions about what is supposed to be happening now.

1) I wonder if I'm eliminating toxins or not. The only thing coming out now is a bright yellow liquid. Also, my tongue is pink. It got a yellowish coating for the first two days, but has since looked pink and normal.

2) I am sick of drinking lemonade. For the past two days, I've only had four cups a day instead of the minimum six. How important is it to keep up the six-drink minimum?

3) In the first three days, I dropped about six pounds, but since then I have not seen additional weight loss. I feel as though I'm at a standstill right now.

I would like to keep going but it's getting harder now that I'm feeling like I've hit a plateau. Thanks for your help!

Peter

Lots of people wonder if they're eliminating toxins or not. The waste comes off in layers. So, you don't see anything happening for days and then have a detox day and see some results. I'd encourage you to continue through the ten days.

If you don't drink the minimum six drinks a day, you won't detox as much. Lots of fluids help to cleanse the kidneys and liver as well as the colon.

Your statement, "I would like to keep going but it's getting harder now that I'm feeling like I've hit a plateau," sounds like a detox day. Let us know how you feel tomorrow.

Person No. 57

I am in my third day of my fast but I feel like I am doing something wrong because I am not seeing much of a change. I decided to go on the fast because I plan on becoming a vegan and wanted to start my new way of life with a cleansed body. The problems that led me to becoming a vegan are my eczema, stomach problems, and back pains. During my fast so far, my stomach has not really hurt. I only feel discomfort right before a bowel movement. Unfortunately, I am still having back pains and I am still scratching my itchy skin. I thought maybe the pain was heightened from all the toxins moving around in my body but I am not sure. The reason I am unsure is because of my BMs.

I apologize if this is TMI (too much information) but I need some help in understanding what is happening to my body. On the first day of my fast, my BM was solid and then runny. On the second and now third I go to the bathroom at least three times, but my BM is small and runny. I don't know if it is because that's all that is in my body. But I think that is not the case because my eczema and back are still acting up. I think I am clogged up and I wanted to know what I could do to clear my system.

I tried drinking the salt water flush but I could not manage it and I am drinking the herbal tea at night and in the morning. Should I try two cups of tea and can I try using one tablespoon of salt in the flush so I can keep it down? Any advice would be appreciated. Thank you.

Peter

Many, myself among them, think the Master Cleanse is the ideal way to begin a move to a healthier diet (only raw fruits, vegetables, nuts and seeds being very, very healthy) as it removes cravings for the processed and cooked foods when it removes the toxins. (See the topic above "Detox Symptoms—Don't Hate Them: They Are Milestones.")

Concerning your situation, the third day is probably too soon to notice big changes if you've never done a cleanse and have been eating meat and cheese most of your life. Big changes usually come after Day 7.

Next, it does sound like you need the salt water flush as well as the tea to move things along. Generally, if you feel like you're clogged up, you probably are. Be sure you're using thirty-two ounces of water and non-iodized sea salt. Then be sure you're only using level teaspoons, not tablespoons. Then try drinking it through a straw. If all that fails, then try your idea of lessening the amount of salt, but don't go all the way down to one teaspoon.

The reason for the salt is to make the weight of the water (scientifically, the specific gravity—this is explained in the "Quick Start" section in Part II) of the water match that of blood so that the kidneys don't absorb the water and the blood doesn't absorb the salt. Then all of it can wash through the system in a dramatic way.

Some people have to drink a few days of salt water before they see a result, so stick with it.

If you have any other questions, just ask. This is a cleanse and the purpose is to eliminate. So these questions about BMs have to be asked and answered so the benefits can be had.

Just continue. It will come out okay in the "end."

Person No. 8
Having done the Master Cleanse once before, I can really say that I feel doing the whole thirty-two ounces of salt water is very important. It does get easier the more your drink it. I can down the whole thing in two minutes, although, when I first get up in the morning the thought of doing it is enough to make me want to go back to bed.

I first got in touch with Peter when I did the first cleanse. I had stopped doing the salt water because I didn't feel it was doing me any good. It just ran right out of me. Peter explained that it is supposed to do that to clean the colon walls. I started doing the salt water again on that cleanse. After being on the cleanse already for a few days, I was surprised as to how much came out. This is after me being on a 90 percent raw food diet (with occasional cheating when going out to a restaurant). So what I am saying is my colon was pretty well cleaned out to begin with.

Over the holidays I ate junk stuff and a little meat and cheese. That food over the six-week period caused my bowels not to move as often as when I got off of the cleanse in November. You should be having a bowel movement after every meal and I was at first. Now on Day 5 of the cleanse my stomach is flat because my colon is really getting cleaned out and I will continue doing the flush after the cleanse because I feel it is very important to keep the colon clean.

A clogged colon is the root of all diseases. If you have never done anything to clean your colon, think about a dirty floor with years of built-up dirt. If you wiped it down you would only get the top layer of dirt so you would have to keep cleaning it. I have been on the Hallelujah Diet since September 2002, and gradually switched to mostly raw this past summer, but it wasn't until I did the Master Cleanse the first time that I felt like my colon was really clean. I had also done several other colon cleansing methods. The Master Cleanse is the quickest, cheapest way to go. Good luck.

Person No. 57
Thank you very much for the response and advice. I will try doing the salt water flush again tomorrow morning. It is Day 4 and I am feeling optimistic. Thanks again.

Person No. 2
I agree with the comments about the salt water flush. Yes, it sucks. Yes, it is awful. Yes, you feel like there is nothing worse you can do to yourself. However, within an hour I have an elimination. That says this stuff works.

I am on my second Master Cleanse. On the first one, I had solid BMs through Day 8. My wife, an RN, didn't believe me. I offered to keep the stuff in the bowl for her to review (joke). She became a believer.

This time (second Master Cleanse) I had one solid BM on Day 3 and one on Day 9. Other than that it looked like salt water mixed with the lemonade. The floor analogy above is a good one. This stuff is coming off/out in layers.

Peter told me that when he eats food that is not good for him, he downs the salt water flush the next morning. I tried that after a red meat day with cheese. For me, it is two or three flushes to get back to feeling good.

Person No.57, I hope you can do the salt water. I think that and a couple of days will start giving you some very tangible signs of improvement. Good luck.

Osteoporosis

Peter

Overeating meat, fat, sugar and processed foods produces an acid condition in the body. This is added to by artificial sweeteners, colors, preservatives and flavors as well as medicines, all of which are treated by the body as acidic toxins. In order to neutralize these, the liver must have alkaline minerals (calcium, magnesium, potassium and sodium). If it doesn't have enough reserves, it must take them from the bones and teeth as the blood must be slightly alkaline. Osteoporosis is the result of taking calcium from the bones. Dental cavities are the result of taking them from the teeth. The current abundance of osteoporosis and concern about calcium is the result of not eating an 80 percent alkaline diet, that is to say, not enough green salads and raw fruits and vegetables.

Other Cleanses—Liver/Kidney/Parasite Cleanse

Peter

Stanley Burroughs, the developer of the Master Cleanse, says it will cleanse all the organs, glands and joints, including the kidneys and liver. People with arthritis have even commented that they noticed joint pain relieved or eliminated. From experience, I know that the Master Cleanse handles many parasites because I have noticed when I pick my nose before a cleanse, I don't afterward. (That is one of the symptoms of parasites. Some of the others being itchy anus, fatigue and overeating.) Other nutritional, natural healers, including Norman Walker, have said parasites require waste accumulations in order to find good breeding grounds. So it makes sense that the Master Cleanse also handles many parasites.

Pain

Person No. 13

Okay, this is my second day on the fast and I am in terrible pain. I'm trying to figure out why and if I will be able to stay on the fast. I really want to.

Yesterday I had a couple of fairly large eliminations. I know this is stuff that's been trapped in there a while. Because of my raw diet I am able to tell what exactly is coming out of me, and this was unrecognizable.

The first one like this was okay. The second one was in the middle of the night last night and I woke up in extreme pain, sweats, etc. After I used the restroom I was able to go back to sleep, but my stomach hurt a while before I could.

Today has been awful. Very, very bad stomach pain and burning. It feels like a lot of stomach acid. I'm familiar with this feeling because my stomach used to overproduce acid. Before I changed my diet, my pH was very bad and my stomach would hurt this way often—just not this badly.

Today I am eliminating a lot of bile and just a little bit of other stuff. The pain seems to subside after I eliminate for a little while, but then it comes right back. I have been too ill to even drink anything yet today, but I am about to try.

I was wondering if anyone has any suggestions on how to combat this horrible pain; if someone else went through the same thing at first; and if so, approximately when it went away. I know it will vary a bit from person to person, but I need some reassurance and to see if this is normal. As much as I want and need to do this fast, I will not be able to if this doesn't start going away. I'm barely able to sit up straight right now and it's definitely interfering with my ability to work. Any suggestions/relative stories would be appreciated.

Person No. 11
Hang in there. I was actually having those symptoms on Days 7 and 8. I don't think it was the senna tea because I was fine with it for the first six days. However, I did experience intense abdominal pain. It felt like something was bubbling in there and I had quite a bit of pain when it was time to eliminate. I also experienced the burning and I could only attribute it to the cayenne since I am eating nothing else! Don't forget that you will have those painful days that normally resolve themselves within the next couple of days. Be sure to drink lots of water. I didn't really drink much because I was so bloated with the lemonade, but now I am making the effort to add extra water. I suppose this first cleanse is a learning period for me. I know for a fact that this will be a lot easier the second time, so hang in there and lots of luck!

Peter
Let's see if we can sort out the pain. Pure senna tea can be too strong and cause a cramping feeling in the abdomen which goes away once the salt water is drunk or lots of lemonade. If that is the case, switch to an herb blend that has senna and other ingredients. Try Get Regular. Drink it only the last thing at night just before you go to sleep. It should take six to twelve hours before it causes eliminations. Sometimes it's

faster. That way your eliminations will be right when you wake up in the morning instead of in the middle of the night.

Interestingly, on my first cleanse, I had very burning BMs from Days 2–7. They do go away. One thing you can do to handle this is drink lots of liquids. Toxins are acidic and apparently you have a lot of them ready to be eliminated. As you continue the cleanse, the lemonade will dissolve these and the BMs will get easier.

Have you taken a lot of medications? Are you overweight? Do you have allergies? All of these are indications of toxicity. More toxicity means the harder the first few days will be relative to others who aren't in that condition. Either way, it gets much easier after Day 5.

Your best course of action is to emphasize the elimination side of the cleanse with drinking lots of lemonade, water, the standard amount of laxative tea and the salt water flush. If it gets to be too much, end the cleanse for now, clean up your diet and do the cleanse again. Remember, getting healthy is not a one-time event. It's a lifetime process.

Person No. 13

Well, as long as I know that it can be normal to have that much pain, I will keep on the cleanse. I am very stubborn. As far as cleaning up my diet goes, I don't think I could possibly clean it up any more. I have been a raw vegan since last June and before that I was a vegan for a couple of months. Now, I realize that the longer I am raw, the better I will feel, but I don't think I can ever reap the full benefits of the lifestyle without doing a cleanse, which is why I am doing one now. Obviously, I have a lot to clean out.

Why? Well, not only did I eat the SAD for 22 years, but worse than that, I am from Louisiana and so therefore I ate the VERY SAD, the Southern American Diet. I ate lots of fried fatty foods, little to no veggies (and those were always cooked and smothered in butter/sugar/you name it), not to mention that I drank nothing but Coke most of my life, tap water when I did have water, used ephedra pills for two years, and did the Atkins diet for a year. Our air quality is very poor. I have breathed in a ton of secondhand smoke. I was never properly fed as a child as my parents never made me eat raw fruits or vegetables and I did not have proper exercise.

All this led to a super case of fibromyalgia which I have had symptoms of since I was about eleven. But at this point I understand it to basically be malnutrition and very bad body pH. I have pretty much conquered it through being raw and juicing greens every day to keep my vitamins and nutrients up and my pH alkaline. The changes have been really amazing and it's really such a simple concept. I wish more people were better educated on these things and willing to make the changes to get healthier.

As far as being overweight, I am 5' 2" and 115 lbs. For myself, (I wish to be 10 percent body fat or less) I probably still have fifteen to twenty pounds of fat to lose. I do have a lot of body fat, no doubt there. All these things would be a good explanation as to why I am so toxic. I anticipate getting rid of it. I'll do anything to be healthier and continue on this path. I will not stop. Thanks for your support. \

Passing Gas—Warning

Peter

I am sorry, but there is no delicate way to say this and IT MUST BE SAID: After you have done the salt water flush for the first time UNTIL YOU COMPLETE THE MASTER CLEANSE, if you feel the need to fart or pass gas, be sure you are on the toilet first. A lot of funny stories result from not following this advice.

Personal Health, Observations on

Peter

1. Each person is responsible for his or her own health.

2. It is wise for a person to learn how to maintain and/or improve their health.

3. Valuable knowledge is available if you take the time to look for it and are willing to determine for yourself whether any knowledge presented is true or false.

4. Each person's body is potentially different. For example, most people find penicillin valuable for killing bacteria. Some people are allergic and die from it.

5. Diagnosis or advice from a health professional is frequently essential, but each person is responsible to determine if it is true or not for his or her own body and whether to follow the treatment.

6. You should use your own good judgment and experience in determining whether to apply the knowledge offered in this book

or on the bulletin board at **www.TheMasterCleanse.com**. Do not accept it blindly. This may mean consulting a health professional.

● Pregnant, Trying to Get

Person No. 12

I've been spotting the whole cleanse. I have had problems getting pregnant, so I think my uterine and girlie organs are repairing themselves. I had a miscarriage last year. I was not producing some hormone that is supposed to double when you're pregnant. Luckily, I lost the baby in the first month. Now the doctor wants to put me on some pills to help me ovulate more. I don't believe ovulating is my problem. I think it's deeper than that. I have been unhealthy for a long time and I think my body can repair itself with this cleanse. I am going to wait to let God do his work. I am going to try for two more months after this cleanse to get pregnant. I'll keep you posted in the months to come.

Person No. 54

I'm on Day 5. This is the second time I've done the cleanse.

My husband and I had been trying to get pregnant for two years. In August of 2002, I quit smoking, then did the five-day MC in September. Lo and behold, in October I discovered I was pregnant. Just an interesting note. The second time is easier, and I'm ready to ride it out until the ole tongue turns pink again, even if that means going beyond ten days. I feel very fortunate that I stumbled on your site. Thanks.

Peter

I recommend two books: *The Wheatgrass Book* by Ann Wigmore, and *Become Younger* by Norman Walker. Both are natural, nutritional methods to improve the general health of the body and therefore pregnancy and children. The following data is from *Pottenger's Cats — A Study in Nutrition* by Francis M. Pottenger, Jr., MD.

From 1932 to 1942, Dr. Francis Marion Pottenger, Jr. conducted an experiment on the effects of heat-processed food on cats.

Dr. Pottenger had an adrenal extract manufacturing company in southern California. At that time, there were no chemical procedures to measure the strength of adrenal extract. So, manufacturers used cats. Cats die without their adrenal glands. So, the amount of extract the cats needed to keep them alive allowed the manufacturers to calibrate the strength of their product. His interest was prompted by the high death rate among his laboratory cats undergoing operations to remove their adrenal glands.

The cats were fed a diet of raw milk, cod liver oil and cooked meat scraps because this was considered the best diet for cats at the time. Concerned with the cats' general health and postoperative survival, Dr. Pottenger noticed the cats had decreased reproductive capacity and that many of their kittens had skeletal deformities and organ malfunctions.

Since this was the middle of the Great Depression and since his neighbors in Monrovia kept sending him increasing numbers of cats they couldn't or didn't want to feed, he couldn't handle the demand for cooked meat scraps. So he ordered raw meat scraps from a local meat packing plant. Always a scientist, Dr. Pottenger fed the raw meat scraps to a separate group of cats so that he could observe any differences between the groups of cats. Within a few months, this group was healthier, their kittens more vigorous, and they had a higher survival rate after their operations.

The contrast between the two sets of cats was so striking, Dr. Pottenger decided to perform a scientific experiment to verify these differences.

The experiment included 900 cats over four generations. The cats were divided into five groups. Each group was supplied with the same basic diet requirements, except for the staple (major part) of the diet. Each group received one of the following staples: raw milk, raw meat scraps, pasteurized milk, evaporated milk or condensed milk.

The raw meat and raw milk groups remained healthy throughout their normal lifespan through all four generations. The first generation of all three processed food groups developed diseases and illnesses near the end of their lives. The second generation of the three processed food groups developed diseases and illnesses in the middle of their lives. The third generation of all three processed food groups developed diseases and illnesses in the beginning of their lives and many died before six months of age. There was no fourth generation in any of the three processed food groups! Either the third generation parents were sterile or the fourth generation cats died before birth. Remember, all four generations of the raw food groups were healthy throughout their normal lifespan.

Is this why so many children are now developing cancer? Why there were no fertility clinics thirty years ago?

There has been no similar experiment ever conducted in scientific literature. The findings were supervised by Dr. Pottenger along with a professor of pathology at the University of Southern California, who was also a pathologist at the Huntington Memorial Hospital in Pasadena.

Protein—a Raw Vegetarian Diet and Weight Lifting

Person No. 1

I am new to the MC way of life. I was curious as to what effect the MC and Stanley Burroughs' recommended nutritional diet would have on a person who lifts weights since Mr. Burroughs' ideas regarding consuming meat for protein are not positive.

Before starting the MC, I ate meat (chicken or fish) once a day and the rest of my meals consisted of raw or steamed veggies and fruit. I would obtain the rest of my daily protein requirement by using protein powders mixed in water. I always ate a balanced protein/carbohydrate/fat ratio as recommended by Bill Phillips (Body for Life). That seems to work for me in balancing my hormones, food cravings and weight control/management.

Question: If I need protein to help repair the muscle I tear down during a lifting session, where am I going to get the needed protein if I am only eating raw/steamed fruits and veggies? (Dairy products are no answer for me as I am lactose intolerant.)

Peter

I am not familiar with Bill Phillips' program, but I can tell you what I have learned about the Master Cleanse and a raw fruit/vegetable/nut/seed diet.

In *The Wheatgrass Book* by Ann Wigmore, she talks about a raw fruit/vegetable/nut/seed diet along with wheatgrass juice as supplying all the needed protein and other nutrients to rebuild the body.

Remember, the largest land animals are vegetarians. They have no trouble building huge muscular bodies with protein. If you feel you need more protein, start adding soaked almonds and seeds to your diet as well. (Soaking the seeds and nuts releases the enzyme inhibitor—the substance that keeps them from sprouting—and makes them easier to digest.)

**The average person needs 30–50 grams of protein a day. That is 1–1.5 ounces per day! In addition, T. Colin Campbell, Ph.D. and nutritional researcher and author of *The China Study*, points out that although meat contains all the essential proteins we need to build our bodies, plants also contain these proteins and by eating an assortment of vegetables we easily meet our protein requirement with proteins that are healthier for us.

For example, spirulina has more than 60 percent protein by weight compared to beef or chicken, which have about 20 percent, which is about the same as sunflower seeds and almonds. Eggs have less than 5 percent, about the same as broccoli and cauliflower.[2]

Victoria and Igor Boutenko, authors of *The Raw Family*, spoke in our area. They said they have seen people lose weight when they first go on an all raw diet and then their bodies rebuild to a healthy weight after some time.

Igor talked about being able to do hundreds of pushups at a time as a result of the body he's rebuilt over many years as a 100 percent raw vegetarian.

To those who wonder if they will get enough protein, Joel Fuhrman, M.D., makes the point in his book *Fasting and Eating for Health* that the average non-overweight person has enough nutrient reserves to fast for at least forty days.

**If you are worried about losing muscle mass when doing the MC, don't. When you stop eating, the liver has enough energy for twelve hours. After that, the body begins to break down muscle to produce needed energy. Two to three days later the body stops burning muscle mass and begins to burn fat, producing a chemical called ketones. Once fat burning begins, muscle mass is preserved and the body begins to literally digest diseased cells, waste and fat.

● Quitting on Detox Days

Peter

In general, don't end your cleanse on a detox day. The Master Cleanse is a rapid form of detoxification so it will usually handle the situation much faster than if you are eating normally. The exception to that is

---

2 *Healing with Whole Foods* Paul Pitchford, p. 143

if you have a detox symptom that hasn't gone away in a few days. If you are experiencing severe detox symptoms and they are not going away after a few days, it may be better to go off the cleanse and slow down the detoxification.

● Running or Exercising During the Diet

Person No. 73
I run approximately fifteen miles per week. Will I need to lay off the running during the cleanse?

Peter
Everyone I know who has done the cleanse has had increased energy. People who do water fasts need bed rest, but not Master Cleansers.

Indeed, I have a friend that runs five miles nearly every day. When he went on a water fast, he had to give up running and could only walk by the fifth day. On the Master Cleanse, he was running all the way up to the twentieth day when he finished the cleanse. Another friend was used to walking four miles a day. On the cleanse he started walking six miles a day and occasionally running a few miles as well! These are not unusual cases. Nearly everyone is surprised to find they have noticeably more energy.

You may occasionally have what I call detox days (usually the second, third, seventh and fifteenth—if you go that long) where you feel tired, irritable or want to eat something solid. However, the symptoms usually pass in a day or two and you feel even better afterward.

Person No. 17
I just want to confirm what Peter said. I work out regularly at the gym. I do one hour on the elliptical machine, which is about five miles. I did this workout with lots of energy on Day 6 of the cleanse.

Also, I provide Swedish massage for a living and on Day 2 I gave three one-hour massages and one hour-and-a-half massage back to back, which is quite a workout and normally would make me quite tired. I felt great afterwards. Again, on Day 5, I did four one-hour massages back to back with lots of energy. I have had much more energy on the MC and without any dips or lows like I usually do at 3:00 p.m. I think you'll find your workout will be no problem and perhaps even better. Good luck!

Person No. 31
I'm on Day 2. At noon, I went to the gym to do my normal routine. I run three miles, do 100 crunches, some arm curls, etc. and had plenty of energy. Overall, I feel great.

Salt Water Flush

Peter
Follow Burroughs' instructions on using sea salt and not table salt. I have heard from a few people who tried using table salt and they told me the taste is very much worse than sea salt. The term sea salt can include those salts that are mined from prehistoric salt beds.

Some people find that drinking the salt water doesn't produce any eliminations for the first couple days. Usually this is true of those who eat meat or dairy products regularly. Adjusting the salt (usually increasing it) does the trick. If you haven't gotten the salt water flush to work by Day 3, switch to another cup of laxative tea in the morning, and try the salt water flush again around Day 8.

Within thirty to sixty minutes after drinking the salt water most people have several urgent, intense eliminations. These generally last for the next 30 to 60 minutes. So, be sure you are close to a bathroom you don't have to wait for during this time. If you are planning on leaving your house, give yourself two hours from the time you drink it until you have to leave the house. If you have had any detox symptoms the previous day, you can expect them to be gone or reduced after these eliminations.

I have found that the salt water flush is easier to do as I go through the cleanse and have less waste in my intestines. Later days are easier than earlier days and later cleanses are easier than early cleanses.

Person No. 58
I did the herbal tea the night before. Then did the SWF the next morning. Why the diarrhea 40 minutes later? It's not explained in the book.

Person No. 18
Are you experiencing diarrhea or is the water just flushing through and taking the contents with it? The purpose of the salt water is to flush your digestive track and take anything present along with it. It normally takes about 45 minutes to an hour for this to happen.

Person No. 13
Yeah, I think a lot of people are mistaking diarrhea with what the cleanse is supposed to be doing.

You're breaking up the old feces and rotten plaque in your intestines. Then you're flushing it through with a lot of liquid. So, yes, the consistency is liquid, and yes, you are seeing brown. But, that is what's supposed to happen. This is cleaning you out.

You're replacing everything you need as far as nutrients and water with the lemonade, so there is no worry of being dehydrated as long as you are drinking enough lemonade.

Person No. 12
I wondered about this also, but it's normal as long as you are not having uncontrollable diarrhea all day long. I still have yet to have a solid mass.

Person No. 13
Yeah, nothing solid here either, which is fine with me. As long as I see something coming out every day, I know it's working.

Person No. 4
I have read the book at least twenty times, but I still have a question. Can I start off with the SWF (salt water flush) this morning if I didn't have a chance to do the herbal laxative last night? My last food consumption was six hours ago and it was just soup. If not, if I do the laxative tea now, how long must I wait to do the SWF?

Peter
The salt water flush should be done only when nothing else has been eaten or drunk before it that day. I learned this the hard way and know of one other person who has done the salt water flush in the middle of the day after lemonade and was quite nauseated.

Also, don't add anything to flavor the water. One person added soy sauce. That is a mistake because soy sauce contains protein, which requires significant digestive work. It is like drinking steak or cooked meat as far as the digestive process is concerned.

Person No. 34

I'm on Day 4 now. I tried the salt water this morning but could only chug down half a quart and then I felt like I was going to throw it all up. So I stopped. I had a tiny BM ten minutes after, but that's it. So, I think I'm just going to stick to the tea. I'm just not having any luck with the salt water. What about anyone else?

Person No. 43

Okay, so I went out and bought the book at my local whole foods today and was so stoked on this whole detox that I went and drank the pint of salt water. Almost immediately, I had a sudden attack of heart burn and had an overwhelming urge to vomit. I'm only nineteen and I'm wondering what could have caused me to be hit with such a violent attack of heart burn. Could it be that I did the salt water flush about an hour after I had eaten?

Peter

Yes, doing the salt water flush after eating is the wrong thing. The salt water flush should be done first thing in the morning after an herbal laxative tea the night before. [By the way, it's a quart of salt water (thirty-two ounces), not a pint (sixteen ounces).]

Person No. 43

In regards to the heartburn I had when I took the salt flush, I think the fact I used two tablespoons instead of two teaspoons caused my horrible discomfort. Today was my first day, too. I intend to try the flush again tomorrow morning.

Person No. 36

This is my first MC and when reading the directions I made note of all measurements. On the first day we did the salt flush first thing in the morning. Apparently I got up too early to try this and instead of using two teaspoons used two tablespoons of salt. Let me assure you that will flush you out quickly and very thoroughly. My wife is still laughing at me.

Person No. 59

I have a question about the salt water flush. Can you drink the salt water flush at night, say around 5:00 p.m., and then take the laxative in the morning? I drive a truck for a living so I work a lot of different hours and it is nearly impossible to do the flush in the morning. In the book it says to take the laxative tea at night and then do the flush in the morning or drink the tea again, but I would rather include the flush.

Peter

The salt water flush should only be done after one wakes up and before any lemonade has been drunk. If you drive during the day, then you will make yourself sick by doing the flush after a day of lemonade. So, you should do another cup of laxative tea instead. My daughter-in-law has done the tea morning and evening rather than the salt water flush and it's produced four or five eliminations a day.

Person No. 13

Well, I just started doing the salt water flush today. The reason I didn't start till today is because I wanted to see how it would affect me, and not on a morning when I had to work. Now I know pretty much what will happen and I can wake up early enough to deal with it properly. I plan to continue doing only the flush in the morning and the tea at night, because the tea seems to be hurting my stomach a lot. I might also try to find another kind. I am currently using Get Regular from Yogi Tea.

Person No. 8

I have a question concerning the amount of salt. I did the normal amount this morning and usually I have a couple of eliminations within the first two hours. This morning I went four hours before any elimination and then it was not very much at all. My question is should I increase the salt or decrease it? Thanks. Also, thanks for the bulletin board. It's fun to keep up on all of the replies.

Person No. 60

I'd like to answer Person No. 8. I think you need to use more salt. The flush should have at least the salinity of sea water. If it is less salty, it is not much different from soup—except for the taste—and soup does not produce eliminations.

It's the salinity of the drink that gives it the laxative effect. I read about traditional sea water enemas in some country that do the same thing, except of course the water is fed from the other end. I have used flushes from common table salt, not sea salt, and it works just as well.

If the SWF doesn't produce eliminations, it is not serious. However, you may find some of your body parts swelling a little. In all the cases I've known, the subsequent flushes produce the eliminations within a few days.

I can think of three reasons why a particular flush didn't work: 1) not enough salt; 2) too much food in the digestive track; or 3) the position of the food in the digestive track. If there is too much food to push to the end, one flush might not be enough. Subsequent flushes will take care of that. The flush works better if food is further down the digestive track. If the flush is done too soon after the last solid meal, it won't work properly. However, these are only problems with the initial flush. After you have been cleaned out, subsequent flushes should be alright as long as the amount of salt is correct.

Years ago, I came across a Japanese fasting method that uses Japanese soy sauce instead of salt. The recipe will make a drink as salty as, you guessed it, sea water. It showed me the flexibility of the system. Now, I use a dash of soy sauce with the salt water to make the drink more appealing. Especially when it's hot, it can taste like salty soup. A good soy sauce can give good flavor.

Peter
**Soy sauce should not be added to the salt water flush. It contains protein (amino acids), which requires significant digestive work. deleted It's like drinking steak or cooked meat as far as the digestive process is concerned.

Person No. 3
I am on day three and I have had no real BMs. Minor ones, but nothing I would consider detoxing. I am using the tea at night and I can only manage half of the salt flush in the morning. I read that increasing the salt might help, but if I can only handle half now, I don't think increasing it will help me. I drink so much liquid, I feel like I am floating. I am not hungry or craving anything. My only detox symptom is a sinus infection. I'm wondering if anyone had any suggestions, or ideas.

Peter
There's hope. Don't despair. First, be sure you're using non-iodized sea salt, not regular white salt. Sea salt is much easier to get down. I recommend Light Grey Celtic Sea Salt. Second, it is not uncommon for people who have been eating meat and dairy products not to have any solid eliminations for the first one or two days. Third, are you drinking laxative tea morning and evening along with the SWF? Until you are eliminating, drink the laxative tea both evening and morning. Once you start eliminating, drink it in the evening only and do only the salt water in the morning.

Person No. 61
Is it normal to feel incredibly thirsty after the salt water flush?

Person No. 74

I am on Day 9 now and have learned that if I wait about thirty minutes after the SWF and drink another thirty-two ounces of water the thirsty feeling goes away. It also seems to help bring on the effects of the SWF super quick. Glad to know it's not just me feeling the thirst.

Sea Salt with Iodine

Person No. 4

I didn't read the label and bought sea salt with iodine added. Is this okay for the salt water flush?

Peter

I recommend that you follow Burroughs' instructions exactly because I know that will produce great results for you. Get non-iodized sea salt. I recommend Light Grey Celtic Sea Salt.

Skin

Peter

Clear skin is an indicator that you are no longer overloading your digestive system with toxins that have to be eliminated. One of the organs of elimination is the skin. When you cease putting cooked food, meat, dairy, artificial colors, flavors and preservatives into your body, your skin clears up quickly as it no longer needs to eliminate "junk," which is what makes your skin look old and ill.

Sleeping Patterns

Person No. 6

Has anyone else's sleeping patterns been disrupted or is it just me? I'm on Day 6 of the cleanse, and although my body actually feels fabulous, I wake up at least two to five times per night to go to the bathroom. Is it the senna or should I stop drinking all liquids at a set time so that I can sleep through the night? Is this just normal? Help! Anybody got any answers out there?

Person No. 1

I did the toilet thing as well. If you did not eliminate that stuff your body would reabsorb the toxins and that would not be good. Do not quit. Just continue with the cleanse.

Peter

You might want to be sure you drink the herbal laxative tea last thing at night as it takes six to twelve hours before it produces results in the early part of the cleanse and faster as you get cleaner. You may also want to switch over to a senna combination tea as senna is pretty strong by itself.

Soy sauce should not be added to the salt water flush. It contains protein (amino acids), which requires significant digestive work. It's like drinking steak or cooked meat as far as the digestive process is concerned.

I discovered that I'd fall asleep much earlier, say around 9:30 or 10:00 on the cleanse and get up around 5:00 to 7:00 a.m.

Person No. 12

I'm on Day 7 and I have no disrupted sleeping patterns, just strange dreams. I actually sleep better and wake up bright-eyed and bushy-tailed!

● Smoking, Quitting During the Cleanse

Person No. 62

I am going to quit smoking January 1st. I am going on the patch. Can I do the cleanse while on the patch? Or should I quit cold turkey while doing the cleanse?

Peter

Burroughs says alcoholics, smokers, and drug addicts on the cleanse find their desire for stimulants and/or depressants goes away.

Person No. 9

Would it be a wise decision to just quit simultaneously with beginning the Master Cleanse? I know that sounds dumb, but it seems harsh to start a fast like that and quit smoking, although it does make sense.

Peter

Never having been a smoker, I cannot answer that except to say that quitting smoking and doing the cleanse has worked well for some.

Try it. If worst comes to worst, you could always go off the cleanse, quit smoking, and then start the cleanse again.

Please let us know what happens as it will be valuable information for others in your "shoes."

Person No. 6

I started the cleanse January 15th. And today is Day 2 for me. I was smoking up to two packs a day and drinking lots of beer. (I know I kept a couple of those companies in business.) At any rate, I decided that was it for me and this is coming from someone who tried to quit smoking at least nine times last year.

I have never experienced a more pleasant time quitting smoking. I think that my mind is so preoccupied with black forest cake, filet mignon and whoppers that I actually don't have much time to think about cigarettes and partying. In all of my fifteen years of smoking, I could never enjoy a cigarette on an empty stomach anyway. Good luck to you! I'm on Day 2 and guess what? I woke up at 5:30 this morning to go to the bathroom and realized something. I wasn't hungry! It just keeps getting easier and easier!

Person No. 61

Does that mean that smoking during the cleanse will severely compromise the results?

Peter

Like the rest of life, it is relative. If you are a smoker and you continue to smoke on the cleanse, your benefits will be less than if you were not smoking. How much less? I do not know. I have heard from smokers that they have gotten good results. If you do want to quit, you will find that it is much easier to quit as the toxins creating the cravings will be speedily eliminated and thus lessen your desires. This may also be true for alcoholics and drug addicts. Burroughs does say it is the case.

Person No. 63

My sister smoked while on the cleanse. Although she was unable to quit smoking, she did get tremendous benefits in other areas from the MC. Smoker or non-smoker, you will definitely benefit from the MC.

Spiritual Breakthrough

Peter

Fasting has been used for thousands of years to produce a temporary heightening of spiritual experience. This is not true for everyone who does the Master Cleanse, but it has happened to some.

Person No. 12

Anyone besides myself have any spiritual encounters?? I had mine on Day 5. I felt Him deep, a feeling so unexplainable that I have never had before. I had uncontrollable streaming tears practically on my knees (weeping), along with some very, very strange coincidences and I don't believe in coincidences. I've always been a believer. I am now convinced about my beliefs and I am in complete bliss!

My first motive for this cleanse was weight loss; it has now changed to a spiritual motive. Let my new journey begin! I'd love to hear some more stories. God bless.

Starvation—Isn't This Starving Yourself?

The only similarity is that both involve no feeding. In his million-copy bestseller, *Fasting, The Ultimate Diet*, Allan Cott, M.D. has 329 citations supporting fasting. 158 are scientific journal articles. He even includes a quotation from *The New England Journal of Medicine*: "Fasting is a valid experience. It can benefit any otherwise healthy person whose calories now have the upper hand in his/her life." In Germany, Japan and Russia, there are annual medical conferences on the benefits of fasting. The 2000 Russian conference heard papers citing the benefits of fasting for treating ten different diseases including asthma, bronchitis, hypertension (high blood pressure), viral lung infections and obesity. The Russian doctor, Yuri Nikolayev, of the Moscow Psychiatric Research Institute was famous for treating 7,000 mental patients successfully with fasting alone after other forms of treatment failed!

Supplements

Person No. 10

I have done the Master Cleanse several times and this time I thought I would add wheatgrass tablets on the evening of Day 4, but cancelled them on the evening of Day 6 as my irritable bowel flared up. Too much fiber?

Peter

Thanks for the info on the wheatgrass tablets. That confirms what Burroughs says about not needing supplements on the cleanse.

By the way, Ann Wigmore, the person who propelled wheatgrass into the public mind, says that either chewing cut, live grass or drinking live, freshly made juice within a few minutes is the only way to use it. She says any form of cooking, drying or storing for a longer length of time reduces its enzymes and life energy to almost nothing. (I just read her book, *The Wheatgrass Book*.)

Surgery and the MC

Because their is no protein on the Master Cleanse, tissue healing or muscle building is reduced. Ask your surgeon by what date he expects you to be healed completely. Then there will be no question about whether you are getting enough protein to heal the operation scar while you are on the cleanse.

Tea, Other Kinds

Person No. 34
I know that occasionally we can drink mint tea to change things, but what about having a cup of green tea or any other type of tea?

Peter
Occasional mint tea and herbal laxative tea in the evening (and optionally in the morning) are the only teas Burroughs lists in his book. When you get to Day 8 or so, you will discover that whatever you went through was worth it.

Person No. 15
It's my second day with the cleanse and everything seems to be flowing smoothly, all puns intended. Thanks for this website. I've found it so very extremely helpful. I have a question concerning teas. I read in a bulletin that organic mint tea is an acceptable extra while doing the cleanse. What about, say, a lemon Rooibos? It's supposed to be very good for you, but I wasn't certain whether all teas are acceptable, or just the laxative and the mint. Any help would be appreciated. I'm going for ten days, wish me luck!

Peter
Hi Person No.15. I am not familiar with Rooibos tea. A search of herbal data on the Internet shows no references to Rooibos being a laxative by itself. There was one mention of Rooibos combined with senna as a laxative blend. That would be acceptable as it contained senna. Other than that, stick with the procedure as written, using an herbal laxative tea or mint tea for variety.

Time Between Cleanses—How Soon Can I Do it Again?

Peter

It is best to space out your Master Cleanses by three or four months and eat lots of fresh greens and salads in between or drink daily green smoothies. You need to build up your calcium, magnesium and potassium reserves because that is what the body uses to neutralize the toxins before they are eliminated. Very rarely (three out of a thousand), a person has done a Master Cleanse every month for several months in a row, which resulted in temporary hair loss. It was handled by taking lots of vitamins and minerals, but it is better to avoid that.

Tingling or Pain in the Teeth

Peter

A very small number of people develop sensitive teeth while on the cleanse. Others have concern about the lemon eating away at their enamel. This is a very rare problem, but for those who have experienced this, it is quite a serious concern. My wife had sensitive teeth on her cleanse and found that drinking lemonade through a straw helped, along with rinsing her mouth after each drink with water (not tap). I believe this ties in with people not having enough alkaline mineral reserves, as the teeth are one place the body can always go to get calcium to neutralize the acidic toxins. Anyone who has sensitive teeth for more than a day on the cleanse should try the straw and rinsing and if the teeth are still sensitive, they should discontinue the cleanse. Then, before doing another cleanse, they should be sure to have lots of greens either in salads and/or green smoothies. See *Green for Life*, Victoria Boutenko's book on green smoothies, for more information and some great recipes.

Tongue Coating

Peter

The coating on the tongue is something Burroughs mentions briefly. He says one of the best ways of knowing when the cleanse is completed is when your tongue is clean and pink. You will discover that it gets very coated during the cleanse. Herbert Shelton, who fasted 35,000 people, says in his book, *The Science and Fine Art of Fasting,* also gives the clearing up of the tongue as one of the two indicators to end the fast. His other indicator is the return of hunger for healthy food.

When I had a furry tongue on the MC, I decided to continue the cleanse until my tongue was clear pink. It took twenty days. A friend did it and it took him twenty-six. The tongue gets coated with white cheezy stuff as you're detoxing. It clears up if you continue. Of course, you can stop the Master Cleanse any time you want, but after the tongue coating is gone you definitely should stop.

Tongue color, shape and coating have been used for thousands of years in traditional Chinese medicine. It is quite amazing all the information that can be learned just from looking at the tongue! A white tongue indicates you are actually eliminating mucus in the intestines. In case you are curious, search on Google for "tongue diagnosis diagram."

Person No. 2
I can vouch for the white tongue thing. I did ten days on my first cleanse and was only starting to get some pink back. I am on my second cleanse and Day 2 is a completely white tongue, headache for twenty-four-plus hours, and the salt water flush is a "pass through" with nothing in it. Last time I did the cleanse, on Day 3 there was an energy boost. I am hoping that will kick in tomorrow. The mint tea has really helped the way my mouth feels.

Person No. 21
This is Day 3 for me. I think things are going normally. I am definitely sleeping more soundly. I usually awaken in the middle of the night, but not the last night. I started the Master Cleanse with a cold and mild asthma, but now the symptoms all seem to be getting better without the use of medication. I think the cayenne is opening everything up.

Usually towards the end of the day I'm dragging badly, but last night I had a lot of pep. I did all kinds of chores and played with my two little boys after dinner.

I'm feeling tired this morning and my tongue is definitely "white." I probably just need to drink some more water. I ordered the MC book yesterday and I'm so anxious to have it. Good luck to all.

Peter
Your white tongue indicates you are actually eliminating mucus in the intestines. The idea of the cleanse is to go until your tongue turns pink again, but not everyone has the time or intention to do it all in one cleanse.

Person No. 2
Day 9. Last two days have been great. I've put in nearly sixteen hour days, six hours of travel one day, lots of "mind" stuff. Tongue is not as pink as I would like, but it is better than MC1 (Master Cleanse the first

time). I've lost eleven pounds as of this morning. I am ready to start back solely on raw food. I am going to only drink juices (got a juicer for Christmas) for about a week. I did not get my Day 7 aches, pains and massive detox like I did in MC1. I don't know if that is good or bad. I am judging just by how pink or not pink my tongue is.

Peter

I'm on Day 10 today and agree with what Person No. 2 said. This time (my fourth Master Cleanse) was much easier. It gets easier and easier. My tongue is nearly all pink! I'm also looking forward to raw food and juices.

I want to add wheatgrass juice to the raw food diet. From what I have read in Ann Wigmore's book, *The Wheatgrass Book*, juicing and wheatgrass are a very important part of four nutritional systems that appear to have helped patients with serious degenerative diseases for decades: The Gerson Institute (juicing, but not wheatgrass), The Optimum Health Institute, The Hippocrates Institute, and the Ann Wigmore Institute.

Peter

For the record, I ended my cleanse on Day 17 feeling great. My tongue went pink around Day 15 and then started to get a light yellowish-grey coating on the back part, but I ended it anyway. There's always another cleanse later. Friends and even strangers notice how healthy and happy I am.

My wife went through Day 15 and felt great also. Her tongue was pink with a light white coat.

I'm now eating raw vegetables, nuts, fruits, seeds, cold pressed olive oil, etc. drinking vegetable juices and experimenting with drinking one ounce of wheatgrass juice a day for a week. So far I've done three days of it. The stuff is vile. You are supposed to, and I have been, sipping it slowly and swirling it around in my mouth before swallowing. The first day it gave me light nausea. It's been a little better since. However, my tongue has gone stark healthy clean pink! I'm continuing my experiment.

Person No. 75

I read that the fast should end when your tongue turns pink again. Does this normally occur around the ten-day mark? I'm planning on doing it for ten days only, but if my tongue hasn't turned by then I guess I keep going?

Peter

For the record, the first time I did the cleanse, I went twenty days before my tongue was completely pink. It took a friend twenty-six days before his turned pink.

You do not have to continue until it is pink. You will still have some great benefits. However, for me and others I know, the wins from continuing until your tongue turns clear pink have included a realignment of priorities and goals, and more spiritual clarity.

Underweight

Peter

When you stop eating, the liver has enough energy for twelve hours. After that, the body begins to break down muscle to produce needed energy. Two to three days later the body stops burning muscle mass and begins to burn fat, producing a chemical called ketones. Once fat is burned, muscle mass is preserved and the body begins to literally digest diseased cells, waste and fat. An extremely underweight friend of mine did the Master Cleanse for more than ten days. She only lost two pounds and those were lost right at the beginning. After the cleanse, she began to put on healthy weight. This same process is described in Allan Cott, M.D.'s second book on fasting, *Fasting as a Way of Life*.

Vegetarian Diet

Peter

As regards moving over to a raw vegetarian diet, I have some suggestions.

Be kind to yourself. Do not beat yourself up if you eat some processed food. Just get back to what you know is healthy. If you find yourself in the SAD rut again, do another Master Cleanse. Each one will help you transition to healthy food more easily. The cravings for processed foods are just coming from toxins that can be eliminated.

Buy and read 12 Steps to Raw Foods by Victoria Boutenko. It will tell you how to live with your friends and family whether they transition with you or not.

Find someone in your area who wants to do this with you. Having a "buddy" makes it doable. I know of several who have wanted to do this and tried, but they failed for lack of support. They had no friends to share stories and recipe experiments.

Finally, please post your experiences, recipes, etc. on The Raw Food Lifestyle board at www.TheMasterCleanse.com for others. We are the beginning of a huge movement toward true vibrant good health—without obscene cost. Thousands will come behind us and go through the same struggles. We can reach out a hand and help them by sharing our experiences, good and bad.

Water Fast Only

Person No. 12

I am on Day 3 of the MC diet and I am doing fine. Is it ok to only have morning bowel movements? I am not going during the day.

I have stocked up on different fasting books to educate myself. One particular book *Fasting and Eating for Health* by Joel Fuhrman, M.D. states that any other fast or diet besides water fasting does not have the same effect or overall benefits as just water. I believe in the MC, but is there more research, studies or books to read about this diet besides Stanley Burroughs or your wonderful site?

Basically, Dr. Fuhrman, who firmly believes in fasting, is saying the organs can not sufficiently detox if you add anything to the water. I am slightly confused. I don't think I could do just water and I don't know how healthy or dangerous this would be.

Person No. 11

I would tend to think the opposite. On a water fast, you are definitely depriving your body of nutrients, whereas on the MC, you do "feed" your body by way of the lemon, syrup and cayenne. Also, don't forget that these ingredients are added because of their added benefits to the detox overall. For example, the cayenne will help loosen up the accumulated mucus, etc. I suppose people have their own preferences. I personally couldn't last on a water fast. I would worry too much about depriving my body of essential nutrients it needs to function properly. Anyway, I hope this helped!

Person No. 12

Thanks for the reply and yes it does help. I agree with you totally. I could never do the water fast. I am on Day 4 and still going strong. The lemonade curbs my appetite and the water fills me up. I look forward to my tea at night, it's like my dessert. It's the salt water, ugh!

Peter

Person No. 11 is right in all he said and I'm glad you're doing well.

The one thing that health and medicine has taught me is that everyone is different. The same antibiotic that cures one will kill another with allergies to it. For the reason that everyone is different, I would say experiment and learn what is best for you. I am not interested in doing a water fast. I know two people who did and they had to have bed rest while they were doing it as they had no energy, but it might be good for your body.

The other thing I know is that more than 90 percent of the people I know who have done this cleanse the way it is written have gotten great benefits.

Weight Loss

Person No. 3
I am extremely interested in the MC. I have done some research on it and I am excited to try it. This week I have found that having a clear reason other than a diet is what keeps one's focus. With that in mind, I have read very little about weight loss and what effect/regaining occurs after the fast is complete, but what about it?

Peter
I was 6' 1" and weighed a little over 230 pounds in June of 2002. I felt terrible, too. My wife had gone on a 100 percent raw vegetable and fruit diet about two months before this. After watching her getting healthier, younger looking and happier, I decided I wanted to feel that way too—even if it meant giving up foods I craved. So, I spent six months eating only raw food and dropped to 198 pounds eating as much raw fruit, vegetables, nuts and seeds as I wanted. Then on January 4, 2003, I started my first Master Cleanse. When I finished it on January 24, I weighed 175 pounds. Four years later, I was eating mostly raw, had done the cleanse several more times and weighed 175.

So you can see that returning to a solid food diet is not necessarily going to make all the weight return. What you eat after you finish your cleanse determines whether you will keep off the weight, continue to lose or put it back on. The cleanse does make me and several others I have heard from want to eat healthier and does remove some cravings for those foods that are bad for your health. I don't feel that people have to give up the "bad" foods completely, just realize they are not daily nutrition, but fun. Keep their consumption in perspective.

Person No. 16
OK, I stopped today after only eight days and I lost thirteen pounds. If I eat 100 percent raw food diet, with fewer nuts than veggies, and fewer veggies than fruit, will I continue to lose weight? It is important to me.

Peter
People lose down to their optimum weight (which is thin) while on a diet that is 100 percent raw veggies, fruit, nuts, seeds, sprouts, etc. Be sure to continue to drink plenty of water: one ounce of water for every two pounds of body weight and more if you are active. Also you need some sea salt each day as well. The cleanse alone won't necessarily make you lose every pound you wish to lose. It is just a good stepping stone.

Person No. 64
Hi. This is my first MC and I am on Day 8. I am following everything (the salt water in the a.m., Smooth Move tea at night and about ten glasses of the lemon drink per day). I have lost about four or five pounds so far. I am about twenty pounds overweight, so I do need to lose weight. Any ideas on why I am not losing much inches or weight? Are there other people that have run into this problem? I am eliminating and I have energy. I appreciate responses.

Person No. 13
**The cleanse alone won't make you lose every pound you wish to lose. It's just a good stepping stone. You must continue after the cleanse by eating more healthy and exercising regularly. There are no shortcuts. This is just a good way to get in the correct mindset for doing these things. The fact that you are eliminating, losing weight, and have energy shows that you are doing the cleanse correctly. Look at the bigger picture. It's doing a lot more for you than just weight loss.

Person No. 64
Thank you for your response. You are correct. I have to concentrate on all the health benefits of the MC. It's just frustrating after not eating for eight days, not to have lost much weight, especially when others are losing ten to fifteen pounds. But, the big picture is important and that is why I went on this cleanse. Thanks for the support.

Person No. 13
You are welcome. You will reach your goals. Just take in a lot more raw fruits and vegetables, and get some exercise in. Start with any exercise

and do it four or five times a week. As you start seeing results you will want to do more and do better. Being healthy is a lifetime process and commitment. It can be fun. It's just a matter of finding what works for you. This is a great motivational tool.

Person No. 65

Hang in there Person No. 64. I didn't lose my weight until Days 11-14 on my last MC and then the third week of raw, the weight really came off. Do not give up now. You have come so far and it's doing your body such good to heal in this way. Stick with it and you'll be so proud of what you've accomplished, no matter what. Take care.

Person No. 64

Thanks, Person No. 65. It's nice to hear that someone else took some time to lose some weight. I actually had only planned on a ten-day cleanse and today is Day 9. Based on what you said about losing at Day 11, I might extend a couple of days, maybe. As you said, the healing benefits are great. Thanks.

Peter

A diet high in meat, fat, sugar and processed foods (the Standard American Diet) will produce an acid condition in the body. In addition, the artificial sweeteners, colors, preservatives and flavors are treated by the body as toxins. What it cannot eliminate, it stores in fat cells. Lose the toxins...lose the fat! When you release the toxins with the cleanse or slower detoxification diet, such as eating only a raw vegetarian diet, the fat is no longer needed as the toxins are gone and the body sheds the fat.

Person No. 16

I'm between twenty and thirty pounds overweight and I am a strict vegan (and aspiring raw foodist). Today was supposed to be the first day of my second cleanse (I stopped two days early a week ago and so I was planning on doing it until the twelfth) but I came home and I couldn't resist the romaine lettuce. I would like to know what you guys think about how much weight I might lose in the next ten days if my diet consists of only laxative tea, our type of lemonade, and romaine lettuce with a light coating of organic soy and vegetable dressing. Thanks for any replies I get.

Person No. 1

I apologize for the long response below but I want to see you succeed with the Master Cleanse,

The Master Cleanse is a total body cleansing program. A few of its side effects are: the removal of internal waste, healthier internal organs, more energy, less toxins stored in the cells of the body, a cleaner, healthier digestive tract, the removal of mucus and hardened plaque from the body which is a precursor for diseases, a better body metabolism, a positive perspective regarding overall health and nutrition, and weight loss.

Speaking from my own experience with the MC, there are no quick fixes and magic pills for obtaining good health and a leaner body. What a person needs is patience, discipline, the right information regarding health and nutrition, wisdom to take this information and apply it properly and, most importantly, determination along with a personal reason that they want to be in better health.

You are on the right track to a healthier body and a better quality of life because you have chosen to do the MC program. I recommend you use the MC program exactly as laid out so you get the positive results you want and follow that with a healthy vegan diet. By doing so, you will lose the weight and keep it off because your body will be free from toxins that cause your liver to not function properly, i.e. a sluggish metabolism.

I decided to do the MC because my metabolism was slow and my hormones were out of balance and I weighed 202 pounds. I was forty years old with adult acne. I walked four miles a day five days a week and I ate no processed foods or high glycemic foods and never lost a pound of weight. Something was wrong with that picture. I picked up a copy of *Natural Awakenings* and read Peter's article regarding the MC and this website.

I did the MC for twelve days. I should have gone longer due to the fact that it was my first time doing the MC. I realized that I have to be patient because one cleanse is not going to undo the effects of the past forty years of poor eating.

To make a long story short, I lost fourteen pounds. I properly broke the fast and am eating raw fruits, veggies and nuts. I have not gained the fourteen pounds back. In fact, I have lost three additional pounds. I took body measurements before starting the MC and my body's proportions have changed. Because I am eating raw fruits, veggies and nuts my body is still detoxing, just very slowly. My metabolism is functioning better than ever. I will do the MC three to four times a year as directed for the rest of my life.

Be patient. So what that you did eight days instead of ten your first time on the MC? Do not beat yourself up over it. Your body still reaped great benefits. Next time it will be a cake walk. Just mentally prepare yourself as to how many minimum days, hopefully ten, you are going to complete and just do it! Trust me. When you meet the goal of ten days you will want to go further. Just monitor your tongue color and listen to your body.

Good luck to you. If my seventy-one-year-old mother and I can do it, so can you.

Women's Issues

Peter

I have received several questions about continuing birth control pills while on the Master Cleanse. I have now heard from several women that they have not had any problems, nor has anyone mentioned any problem.

Person No. 16

I had my period two weeks ago. I started again today, Day 1 of the cleanse. Is the cleanse to blame?

Person No. 66

It probably is the cleanse causing a flushing of the system. I have read that the body uses the period to cleanse itself. I found that when I do a major cleanse or change in diet that sometimes my period comes on sooner than expected.

If the flow is a normal one, there shouldn't be a cause to worry. If it is heavy, but you are not feeling tired, a lack of energy or weak due to the heavy flow, then also, don't worry.

Person No. 12

I have a very important question. I've been looking all around the web and can't find answers. I have been spotting this whole fast. I have never spotted in between periods ever. They are usually right on time. I had an ectopic pregnancy [pregnancy outside the uterus in the tubes] due to scar tissue in the tubes and a miscarriage from not producing some hormone.

Yesterday on Day 12, I experienced major, major cramps in my uterus. I don't know if it was me ovulating (sometimes I can feel it), but it was horrible. I also read it could have been gas in the uterus. I feel better today and had a semi-solid movement this morning. I am breaking the fast with fruit today.

Am I shedding my uterine walls? Can the scar tissue be releasing? Is this common? Do you think gas? I am still spotting this morning. I experienced these major pains while at work sitting upright. When I got home last night and laid down I felt ok. After my bowel movement I felt good too. Was it the colon pushing on my uterus? Help! Any websites, testimonials, books, etc., etc. will help.

Peter

You will have to seek a professional or look within yourself. I believe firmly that every person knows the truth when they see or hear it. There is something in us that responds to truth, much like one guitar string starts to vibrate when another one is vibrating close by it. Along those lines, I will give you some of my thoughts, which I hope will help.

Numerous women have reported that the Master Cleanse influences periods in several ways. Initially it may produce spotting or premature periods. This is because a woman's periods are a detoxification process. Occasionally it may bring on an extended period. Generally, by the end of the cleanse it tends to normalize periods and make them easier, the idea being that it is the toxins that make periods difficult.

I believe that the spotting and cramps might have been due to the detox of your uterus, which may have been denied the proper nutrients and adequate supply of clean, pure blood for many years. Such a condition would have been brought about by years of very bad diet and no cleansing and could have been the reason for your ectopic pregnancy.

When someone detoxifies, she often turns on conditions brought about by toxins as the toxins are eliminated on the cleanse. It is not uncommon for people with histories of rashes to turn on a rash for a day or two while on the cleanse before the rash goes away.

If your problems don't go away after a couple days off the cleanse, I would see a doctor. If they do go away, you might want to consider putting yourself on a health-restoring regimen for several months.

I believe such a regimen should include:

1) Not filling the body with more toxins as found in refined white flour and sugar products; meat; artificial flavors, colors, preservatives; alcohol; tobacco; dairy products, etc.

2) Detoxifying the colon to eliminate the toxins being reabsorbed by the blood and redistributed throughout the entire body. (The Master Cleanse is a way of doing this.)

3) Ensuring the body gets adequate good (non-tap) water (at least one ounce daily for every two pounds of body weight); non-iodized, unprocessed sea salt; and nutritional, raw vegetables (especially greens), fruits, sprouts, and soaked seeds and nuts to help the body rebuild the depleted nutritional reserves and organs.

4) Removing any stress-producing situations in the current environment.

5) Getting exercise and fresh air by lots of walking.

I was once giving a speech in a health food store and a woman in her mid-twenties came up and asked to speak to the group. She said she had never met me, but wanted to thank me because she had fibroid tumors which disappeared during a Master Cleanse, which she started because she read my book.

I found an interesting article on the Web by J. Kunjufu, Ph.D., who points out that poor diet can lead to fibroid tumors. In addition to direct problems, such as heavy bleeding and tremendous pain, they can over time result in backache, kidney obstruction and even miscarriages. Among his recommendations to resolve or prevent these, he suggests fasting for one to three weeks; eating a vegetarian diet; drinking wheatgrass juice; exercise; daily enemas; herbs; removing cooked food, meat and dairy products from the diet; meditation and prayer.

Person No. 12
It helps a great deal, thank you. The article was helpful too.

The pain has gone. I will continue the salt water thing you suggest, good diet etc. I appreciate everything. I'm going to try to cross over to a vegetarian diet.

Word of mouth

From 1976 to 2004, the Master Cleanse spread by word of mouth alone. An informal survey I did in 2005 of 141 people who had done the Master Cleanse revealed that, on average, each person who does it inspires at least three more people to try it. That is pretty impressive. I know when I finished my first Master Cleanse I certainly wanted to tell the world, which I did from my website, **www.TheMasterCleanse. com. Within four months, I had more than a thousand people visit and in January 2004 had 100 people doing the Master Cleanse on the website's bulletin board. I personally answered every question for the entire month.

From this I learned several things. Most important was that verbal directions are like playing telephone. You remember? You whisper something to someone who whispers what they heard to someone else, etc. down the line through several people. The message is NEVER the same. For example, I have been told that each day you eat vegetable soup; that eating fish was part of the Master Cleanse; and that each lemonade drink contained 32 oz. of water. I have talked to people who were surprised to hear about the salt water flush and laxative tea as they weren't told about it! I think you get the idea.

I want you to get the best possible results. That comes from doing exactly what Stanley Burroughs developed. If you do not know what that is, you cannot be sure you are going to get the results you want. Please when you get great results and want your friends to get the same, ensure they do by telling them to get either *The Master Cleanser* by Stanley Burroughs, this book, or the "Master Cleanse Coach iPhone app" by Peter Glickman. Then they will have the correct information.

Afterword

Before time, there was and is understanding, peace, compassion, awe and bliss. Good health is a reflection of that and as such cannot be separated from it, no more than you could separate the reflection of a flower from the mirror.

When we hurt, feel depressed or seem cut off from that understanding, peace, etc., it can only be because we have chosen to use our limitless power to conceal the ultimate truth from ourselves.

Joyously, the reverse is also true. Desiring, seeking, observing and acting are the keys which will always unlock our self-made prison door.

This book is dedicated to you and your good health.

References

Anderson, Richard, N.D. (Doctor of Naturopathy: Teaches patients to use diet, exercise, lifestyle changes and natural therapies to enhance their bodies' ability to heal itself), *Cleanse & Purify Thyself Book 1.5*, Triumph Business, 1998

Airola, Paavo, Ph.D., N.D., *How to Get Well*, Health Plus Publishers, Phoenix, AZ, 1974

Barile, James J., N.D., D.C. (Doctor of Chiropractic: Uses manipulation by hands to unblock nerve flow to allow the body to heal itself), Ph.D., *Why Didn't Someone Tell Me Sooner? A How-to Guide for the Restoration & Maintenance of Health*, Autumn Press, Feura Bush, NY, 1997

Bieler, Henry G., M.D. *Food is Your Best Medicine*, Ballantine Books, New York, NY

Boutenko, Victoria, *Green for Life*, North Atlantic Books, Berkeley, CA, 2010

Boutenko, Victoria, *12 Steps to Raw Foods*, North Atlantic Books, Berkeley, CA, 2007

Bragg, Paul, *The Miracle of Fasting*, Health Science, Santa Barbara, CA, 2004

Burroughs, Stanley, *The Master Cleanser*, Burroughs Books, Reno, NV, 1976

Burroughs, Stanley, *Healing for the Age of Enlightenment*, Burroughs Books, Reno, NV, 1976

Campbell, T. Colin, Ph.D., *The China Study: Startling Implications for Diet, Weight Loss and Long-Term Health*, BenBella Books, Dallas, TX, 2004

Cott, Alan, M.D., *Fasting—The Ultimate Diet*, and *Fasting as a Way of Life*, Hastings House, Norwalk, CT, 1997

Ehret, Arnold, *Rational Fasting*, Ehret Literature Publishing Co., Dobbs Ferry, NY, 1994

Fuhrman, Joel, M.D., *Fasting—and Eating—for Health*, St. Martin's Griffin, New York, NY, 1995

Fuhrman, Joel, M.D., *Eat to Live,* Little, Brown and Company, New York, NY, 2005

Haas, Elson, M.D., *The New Detox Diet: The Complete Guide for Lifelong Vitality with Recipes, Menus, & Detox Plans,* Celestial Arts, Berkeley, CA, 2004

Hubbard, L. Ron, *Clear Body, Clear Mind,* Bridge Publications, Inc., Los Angeles, CA, 1994

McCoy, Frank, M.D., *The Fast Way to Health, 11th ed.* (Originally published 1926), published as an eBook by Peter Glickman, Inc., 2009

Pottenger, Jr., Francis M., M.D., *Pottenger's Cats,* Price-Pottenger Nutrition Foundation, La Mesa, CA. 1983

Shelton, Herbert M., *The Science and Fine Art of Fasting,* Natural Hygiene Press, Chicago, IL, 1978

Walker, Norman, D.Sc. (Doctor of Science: in the US equivalent to Ph.D., in foreign countries advanced degree beyond Ph.D.), *Colon Health: The Key to a Vibrant Life,* Book Publishing Co., Summertown, TN, 1995

Walker, Norman, D.Sc., *Become Younger,* Book Publishing Co., Summertown, TN, 1995

Wigmore, Ann, *The Wheatgrass Book,* Avery, New York, NY, 1985

Index

A

acids
 acidic foods, 112, 127–128, 154
 amino acids, 141, 143
 bile, 59
 lemons, 22, 31, 45–46
 Pantothenic Acid (B5), 94
 toxins, 14, 28, 54–55, 91, 129, 147
 uric acid, 13
addictions, 20, 27, 91–92, 143–144.
 See also smoking
agave nectar, 23, 48, 110
agitator and rinse cycle, 27, 31–32,
 40–41
alkalinity
 blood, 118, 123
 teeth, 19–20, 94, 128, 147
 toxins, neutralizing, 14, 22, 45–46,
 91, 130
allergies, 30, 33–34, 116, 130
alternative medicine
 Chinese, 51, 147–148
 healing crises, 28–29
 naturopathy, 4, 96, 116
anti-aging, 9–13
antibiotics, 25, 34
anti-depressants, 26, 42, 49, 115–117
arthritis, 9–10, 72, 128
asthma
 children and, 33
 detox concerns, 85
 fasting as treatment for, 65, 86, 93,
 145, 148
Atkins diet, 22, 57–58, 60–61, 130
autointoxication, 5

B

bentonite, 35, 49–51, 119
berries, 64
bile, 59–60, 72, 89, 129
birth control pills, 156
blood. *See also* high blood pressure

alkalinity, 118, 123
 blood sugar, 19, 25, 26, 88, 93,
 109
 blood thinners, 34, 116, 117
 cayenne affecting, 17, 23, 31,
 68,115–116, 123
 cooked foods affecting, 30, 107
 hypoglycemia, 95
 lactose, 81
 salt water flush, 21, 126
 toxin reabsorption, 29, 31, 157
Blood Type Diet, 111
Body for Life (Bill Phillips), 134
boredom, 27, 52–53, 78, 98–99
Boutenko, Victoria, 30, 107, 135, 147,
 150
bowel movements
 bentonite and psyllium, 35, 49–51,
 119
 burning, 28, 54–55, 82, 84, 129–130
 after cleanse, 24, 65
 color changes
 black, 35, 77
 yellow, 30, 55, 59–61, 72, 112,
 124
 delayed, 22, 35–36, 57–58,61–63,
 120–121,141
 dependency on salt water flush,
 102
 irritable bowel syndrome, 25, 145
 in layers, 29–30, 41, 56, 58–59, 74,
 112, 124, 127
 in the mornings, 27, 40, 75, 95, 102,
 129, 151
 runny, 20, 55–59, 69, 88–90, 125,
 137–138
 tiredness, 77
breastfeeding, 33, 113
breaking the cleanse
 gas, 25
 nausea, 24
 orange juice, 25, 96, 114

breaking the cleanse *(continued)*
  soup, 18, 25, 63–65, 114
Burroughs, Stanley, x

C
caffeine, 28, 29, 35, 40, 91–92
calcium
  alkalinity, 19–20, 46, 91, 128
  in maple syrup, 94
  neutralizing toxins, 146, 147
calories, 6–7, 9–12, 39, 108, 145
cancer. *See also* chemotherapy
  age-related, 9, 10
  avoiding, 6
  children and, 133
  fluoride as cause, 16, 70
  prevalence, 2, 4
  excess protein as cause, 15
candida, 24, 66
Carrel, Alexis, 12
Cascara Sagrada, 102
cats, nutritional experiments on,
  132–134
cayenne pepper
  acquired taste, 24, 35, 67, 76, 121
  amounts, 16, 18, 22, 26,120
  affecting blood, 17, 23, 31, 68,
  115–116, 123
  burning sensation, 28, 129
  capsules, 17, 68, 122
  cramps, relieving, 74
  heat increase, 39, 68, 103–104
  minerals, providing, 118
  mucus, dissolving, 23, 68, 115, 123,
  148, 151
  waste, dissolving, 56, 80, 119
  website link, 67
cheating, 68, 69, 84, 85, 108, 122
chemotherapy, 32, 34, 42, 70, 116
chewing, desire for, 27, 69, 71, 79
chicken heart, 12–13
Chinese medicine, 51, 147–148
cigarette smoking. *See* smoking
circulation. *See* affecting blood *under*
  cayenne pepper
cold, feeling, 58, 72–73
cold turkey, 28, 35, 143
colon
  Atkins diet clogging, 22
  colonics, 43, 73–74, 119

colon *(continued)*
  dairy clogging, 56, 59
  diseases, 127
  detoxifying, 29, 123, 125, 157
  meat, clogging, 22, 31, 57
  mucus in, 81
  probiotics, 65
  psyllium, 49–51, 119
  salt water flush, 61, 112, 126
  senna as harsh on, 102
  uneliminated waste in, 5, 31
constipation. *See* delayed *under*
  bowel movements
cooking for others, 38, 40, 75, 78, 84
Cott, Allan, M.D., 7, 14, 51, 145, 150
cramping. *See also* bowel movements
  cayenne easing, 74
  detox causing, 77, 79, 156–157
  from senna tea, 20, 55, 56, 89, 96, 129
cravings
  Body for Life (Bill Phillips) easing,
  134
  for caffeine, 92
  for cigarettes, 144
  detox symptom, 30, 68, 74–75, 98,
  99, 122
  eased by eliminations, 27, 29, 37
  healthy foods, 46, 56, 152
  hunger, 39, 79, 89, 94–95
  for maple syrup, 108–109
  probiotics easing, 24, 47
  for Standard American Diet, 77,
  125, 150
Crohn's disease, 50
cycles, seven day, 30–31, 38

D
dairy
  colon, clogging, 56, 59
  delayed eliminations, causing, 22,
  60–61, 137, 141
  drinking after cleanse, 46–47
  milk, 20, 74, 133
  not recommended, 13, 111, 158
  as toxic, 27, 29, 81, 142, 157
depression, 6, 93, 118
Detox Diet Scale, 42–43
detoxification process, 37
detoxification symptoms. *See also*
  toxins

Index

detoxification symptoms *(continued)*
  boredom, 27, 52–53, 78, 98–99
  burning bowel movements, 28,
    54–55, 82, 84, 129–130
  cravings, 30, 68, 74–75, 98, 99, 122
  irritability, 27, 30, 37, 99, 136
  nausea, 24, 28, 63, 65, 138, 149
  rashes, 29, 37, 80–81, 101, 157
  severe, 22, 29, 30, 33–34, 49, 83, 135
  sinus infections, 86, 141
  tiredness, 27, 29, 37, 80, 90, 136
  as unpleasant, 26–27
  vomiting, 28, 62, 65, 81, 110, 139
diabetes
  increasing, 3
  as frequent cause of death, 4
  as disease of old age, 9, 10
  special instructions, 25–26, 88,
    94,114
diet pills, 95
diarrhea. *See* runny *under* bowel
  movements
digestion, 24, 31, 71
DNA damage, 10
dreams
  of accomplishment, 54, 58, 89
  of cheating on cleanse, 69
  strange, 120, 143
  triggering fears, 89
drug addiction, helped by cleanse,
  27, 143–144

E
Edison, Thomas, 15
eczema, 86, 125
enemas, 43, 140, 158
energy
  digestion, 24, 31, 71
  lack of, 6, 27
  increased by cleanse, 19, 90, 106,
    136, 154
  supplied by maple syrup, 23, 94
  muscles, 32, 41, 135, 150
enzymes, 86, 125
Epsom Salt, 30, 34, 43, 70
exercise
  after cleanse, 153
  during cleanse, 33, 43, 53, 90, 134,
    136
  naturopathy, 4, 5, 96

F
Fasting as a Way of Life (Cott), 7, 14,
  150
Fasting Can Save Your Life (Shelton),
  95–96
Fasting, The Ultimate Diet (Cott), 7,
  14, 51, 145
fatigue, 6, 27, 29, 37, 80, 90, 136
fertility, 12, 133
fibromyalgia, 109, 130
flax seeds, 49
fluoride, 16, 24, 66, 70, 121
fruits
  alkalinity, 45, 128
  bowel problems, easing, 5–6
  after cleanse, 46–48, 51, 63–64, 88
  for breaking cleanse, 18, 25
  as detoxifiers, 43, 83, 99, 155
  lacking in Standard American
    Diet, 61, 130
Fuhrman, Joel, M.D., 73, 90, 96, 135,
  151

G
gas, 25, 48, 71, 131, 156–157
grapefruit juice, 25, 65, 96, 114
green smoothies, 19, 43, 65, 146, 147
Green for Life (Boutenko), 147
gum, chewing, 39, 71

H
Hallelujah Diet, 51, 127
hair loss, temporary, 19, 91, 147
headaches
  caffeine withdrawal causing, 28,
    29, 35, 40, 91–92
  during cleanse, 69, 96, 99, 100, 148
  excess protein causing, 15
health care, 2–3 , 7–8
heart disease, 2–3, 4, 10, 11, 15
heartburn, 139
hemorrhoids, 28, 81, 93
Herxheimer Reactions, 28
high blood pressure
  borderline, 11
  cause of death, 2, 4
  disease of old age, 9
  fasting effects, 11, 65, 93, 116, 117,
    145

high blood pressure *(continued)*
  obesity, 3
  special instructions, 25–26, 34
high fructose corn syrup (HFCS),
  27, 48
honey, 93–94
hunger
  confused with cravings, 39, 79, 89,
    94–95
  during cleanse, 11, 37, 69, 97, 147
hypoglycemia, 95

I
infertility, 95–96
intestines. *See* colon
irritable bowel syndrome, 25, 145
irritability, 27, 30, 37, 99, 136

J
juices. *See also* orange juice
  grapefruit, 25, 65, 96, 114
  sugar cane, 22, 23, 94, 108, 110–111
  wheatgrass, 51, 134, 145, 149, 158
junk food. *See* Standard American
  Diet

K
kidneys
  calorie reduction aiding, 7
  cleanse aiding, 72, 77, 128
  fluids cleansing, 123, 125
  salt water flush, 126

L
lactose intolerance, 81, 134
Lane, William A., Sir, 4–6
lemons
  amount for cleanse, 16, 18, 22–23,
    26, 35, 98, 104
  bottled juice, 17, 22, 35, 42, 103, 105,
    120
  enzymes in, 17, 22, 40, 42, 103, 105
  acid/alkaline nature of, 45–46
  organic, 22, 54, 104–105, 106, 121
  squeezing methods, 105
lemonade
  blood sugar, keeping level, 95
  cayenne, 23–24, 67–68, 123
  cramps, relieving, 20, 56, 96, 129
  dehydration, preventing, 138

lemonade *(continued)*
  drinking after ending cleanse, 25,
    47, 64, 107
  finishing two hours before bed,
    102–103
  heating, 73
  hunger, eliminating, 39, 94–95 ,
    151
  premixing, 22–23, 39, 103
  pulp, 104–105
  purified water, using, 16
  salt water flush, drinking after 18,
    20–21, 138, 139
  six-drink minimum, 16, 26, 38, 92,
    98, 122–124
  straw, drinking through, 124, 147
  sweetness, reducing, 88, 112
  toxins, dissolving, 130
  waste, loosening, 31, 35, 40, 48,
    58, 83
limes
  as alternative to lemons, 18, 22, 26,
    39, 71, 104, 114
  organic, 16, 106
  pasteurized, 17
liver
  alkaline minerals,128
  calorie restriction, 7
  chemotherapy, 32
  fluids aiding, 123, 125
  high fructose corn syrup (HFCS),
    48
  liver cleanse, 71–72, 73, 77
  toxins in, 14, 32, 46, 155

M
Madal Bal syrup, 107
magnesium
  as alkaline mineral, 91, 128
  in maple syrup, 94, 118
  neutralizing toxins, 19, 46, 146
maple syrup
  agave nectar no substitute, 48,110
  amount for cleanse, 18, 22, 26,
    108–109
  cravings for, 108–109
  energy supplied, 23, 94
  as expensive, 17, 105
  honey no substitute, 93–94
  Madal Bal Syrup no substitute, 107

Index

maple syrup *(continued)*
  molasses substitute, 88
  nutrients in, 39, 48, 59, 94, 118
  organic grade B or darkest, 16, 23, 88,
  reducing amount, 23, 112, 108, 110–111
  sorghum substitute, 23, 110
  sugar cane juice substitute, 23, 94, 108, 110
  yeast, 66
MasterCleanse.com, The, *See under* www.TheMasterCleanse.com
Master Cleanser, The (Burroughs), *x*
meat
  acid producing, 45, 127–128, 154
  breaking-cleanse soup, not part of, 18, 25, 63
  after cleanse, 47, 127
  clogging colon, 22, 31, 57
  craving, 27, 46
  delaying cleanse effects, 35, 56, 59–61, 125, 137, 141
  in Pottenger cat experiment, 133
  not recommended, 13, 29, 134, 157–158
  toxin producing, 81, 142
  for weight control, 111–112
medications
  anti-depressants, 26, 42, 49, 115–117
  blood thinners, 34, 116, 117
  for constipation, 36,120
  continuing during cleanse, 18, 21, 34, 51, 116
  causing severe detox symptoms, 83
  dose affected by fasting, 11, 26, 93, 117
  high blood pressure, 11, 26, 34, 93, 116–117
  medical drugs as toxins, 30, 81, 115, 130
menstruation, 105, 156–157
metabolic waste, 12, 13
metabolism, 73, 123, 155
milestones, 28–30, 76, 125
milk, 20, 74, 133 *See also* dairy
miscarriages, 132, 156, 158
molasses, 26, 88, 94, 108

mood improvement
  later in cleanse, 19, 27, 31, 52, 79, 100
  proper nutrition leading to, 105
mucus
  bentonite and psyllium removing, 49, 51
  cayenne pepper dissolving, 23, 68, 115, 123, 148, 151
  flakes, 55
  as form of protection, 47, 81, 87
  salt water flush, 21, 40
  white tongue, 148
mucoid plaque, 118–119
muscles, 32, 41, 135, 150

N
naturopathy, 4, 5, 96, 116
nausea, 24, 28, 63, 65, 138, 149
Natural Awakenings, 106, 116, 155
Neera Super Cleanse, 107
nuts
  alkalinity, 45
  after cleanse, 47, 51, 64, 69, 88
  part of health-restoring regimen, 29, 125, 158
  soaking for easier digestion, 134

O
obesity. *See also* Standard American Diet
  increasing in US, 3
  as cause of death, 4
  fasting treatment, 65, 93, 145
  sign of toxicity, 30, 34, 122, 130
  high-fructose corn syrup causing, 48, 23
organic products
  expensive, 105
  flax seeds, 49
  lemons, 22, 54, 104–105, 106, 121
  maple syrup, 16–18, 23, 88, 108, 110–111
orange juice
  after the cleanse, 18, 25, 63–65, 96, 114
  grapefruit juice alternative, 25, 65, 96, 114
  prohibited during cleanse, 37
osteoporosis, 15, 20, 128
overweight. *See* obesity

P

pain. *See also* cramping
  back pain, 78, 125
  burning eliminations, 28, 54–55, 82, 84, 129–130
parasites, 50, 77, 128
patch, the, 143
Phillips, Bill (*Body for Life*), 134
pitfalls, 36–40
plateaus, 29, 124–125
potassium
  alkalinity, 19, 91, 128
  in maple syrup, 48, 94
  neutralizing toxins, 46, 146
Pottenger, Jr., Francis M., M.D., 132–134
prayer, 53, 158
pregnancy and cleanse, 33, 132
probiotics, 16, 19, 24–25, 47, 65
protein
  animal sources, 13, 112, 134–135
  children and, 33
  cleanse lacking, 32, 43, 90, 145–146
  deficiency symptoms, 14
  endotoxins, 5
  excess symptoms, 15
  soy sauce, 36–37, 138, 141, 143
psyllium, 35, 49–51, 119

Q

quick start instructions, 17–18

R

rashes, 29, 37, 80–81, 101, 157
Raw Family (Boutenko), 135
rinse and agitator cycle, 27, 31–32, 40–41
running, 90, 136

S

SAD. *See* Standard American Diet
salt water flush. *See also* sea salt
  blood, same weight as, 21, 126
  colon health, 61, 112, 126
  diarrhea, 20
  delay in eliminations, 21, 35, 57, 61
  detoxifying, 28, 30, 34, 91
  eliminations, 21, 55, 82, 83, 88, 112

salt water flush *(continued)*
  heartburn, 139
  dependency on, 102
  in the mornings, 61, 68, 70
  mucus, 21, 40
  occasional flushes, 47, 52
  as rinse cycle, 27, 31–32, 41
  adding soy sauce to, 36–37
  on empty stomach, 22, 47
  substituting laxative tea, 101, 112
  tiredness, causing, 27
  not tolerating, 62, 83, 86, 111
  purified water recommended, 16
Science and Fine Art of Fasting, The (Shelton), 12, 13, 147
Schulze, Richard, 17, 68
Schultz herbal cleanse, 51
sea salt
  Light Grey Celtic, 21, 141–142
  non-iodized
    as part of healthy living, 29, 153, 158
    as part of shopping list, 16, 111
    verses table salt, 20–21, 62,112, 137, 141–142
  recommended amounts for cleanse, 18, 20–21, 35–36, 44, 71, 120, 126
  sparing use of in vegetable soup, 18, 25, 63
seeds
  after cleanse, 47, 49, 51, 64, 69, 88
  alkalinity, 45
  health-restoring regimen, 29, 125, 158
  soaking for easier digestion, 134
senna. *See under* teas
seven day cycles, 30–31, 38
Shelton, Herbert, 12–13 , 95–96, 147
skin improvement
  blemishes, 41, 78–79, 83–84, 88, 97
  detoxification sign, 75, 76, 112, 142
  dryness disappearing, 101
sleep, cleanse affecting, 79, 88, 142, 143, 148
smell, sense of
  food, 42, 52, 77, 99, 100
  heightened, 41, 76, 78, 79, 97
smoking, 27, 57, 77, 132, 143–144
sorghum, 23, 94, 110

soup. *See also* vegetables
 breaking the cleanse, 18, 25, 63–65, 114
 broth, 87–88
 chicken broth, 113
 during the cleanse, 37, 39, 75
soy sauce, 36–37, 138, 141, 143
spiritual experience
 breakthrough, 53, 90, 97, 105, 144–145
 in later part of cleanse, 19, 52, 100, 101, 106, 150
spirulina, 135
sprouts. *See* seeds
Standard American Diet (SAD)
 acid condition, creating, 154
 backup, causing, 82
 cravings, 77, 125, 150
 defined, 61, 130
 mucoid plaque, 119
 overweight, causing, 122
 results of cleanse, delaying, 120
straws, drinking liquid through, 21, 62, 112, 124, 126, 147
stress, 4, 29, 52, 84–85, 90, 100, 158
stomachaches. *See* cramps
sugar. *See also* blood sugar *under* blood
 as acidic, 45, 127, 154
 reducing calcium, 19–20
 in maple syrup, 23
 not recommended, 29, 43, 88, 157
sugar cane juice, 22, 23, 94, 108, 110–111
supplements, 17, 39, 118, 119, 145
sweeteners, artificial, 109, 127, 154

T
teas
 Get Regular, 20, 129, 140
 green, 146
 mint
  freshening breath, 66, 111, 148
  adding sweeteners, 109–110
  unlimited amounts allowed, 18, 26
  water alternative, 24, 36, 69, 71, 114, 120
 Rooibos, 146
 sarsaparilla, 114–115

senna
 blended, 16, 56, 96, 101–102, 111–112, 146
 causing cramping, 20, 121, 129
 serving limits, 32, 49–50, 59
 strong, 115, 142
Smooth Move
 combination tea, 20, 112
 senna-containing, 101, 111, 121
 taken in the evening, 124, 129, 153
Yellow Dock, 121
teeth
 alkaline levels, 19–20, 94, 128, 147
 brushing during cleanse, 46, 66, 111
temptation, 53, 73
TheMasterCleanse.com, The, *See under* www.TheMasterCleanse.com
thirst, 141
tiredness, 6, 27, 29, 37, 80, 90, 136
tongue
 coated, 19, 46, 79, 85, 124, 147–149
 pink, 72, 76, 86, 132, 150
 as diagnostic tool, 51–52, 66, 92, 148, 156
toxins. *See also* detoxification symptoms
 as acidic, 55, 94, 127–128,129–130,147
 agitator and rinse cycle, 31, 41
 bowel movements, 54, 57, 124, 125, 142
 cancer patients, 70
 cleanse relieving, 50, 56, 121, 142
 cravings, 75, 77, 98, 125, 144, 150
 endotoxins, 5
 Epsom Salt baths drawing out, 34
 stored in fat, 122, 154
 toxic foods, 29, 157
 chewing gum as toxic, 71
 headaches, 91
 medications, 93, 115–116
 menstruation, 157
 metabolic waste, 13
 sluggish metabolism, causing, 155
 mucus, 81, 86, 87
 need for neutralization, 14, 19, 46, 91, 146

toxins *(continued)*
  older toxins, 35, 41
  reabsorption into blood, 29, 31, 157
  symptoms of toxicity, 33–34
  weight gain, causing, 47–48
  yeast as toxin, 66
Twelve Steps to Raw Foods (Boutenko),
  150

U
underweight, 150

V
veganism
  alternating vegan diet with cleanse,
    107
  vegans on cleanse, 81, 85, 111, 121,
    130, 154–155
  vegan diet as detoxifier, 43
vegetables. *See also* soup
  alkaline minerals, 14, 45
  bowel problems, answer to 5–6
  detoxifying, 83, 99
  greens emphasized, 29, 158
  as healthy, 51, 64, 69, 88, 107, 125
  juice, 43, 47, 149
  osteoporosis, preventing, 128
  proteins, 134–135
  vitamins in, 43, 130
  for weight loss, 47, 112, 152, 153
vitamins
  B vitamins and urine color, 59–60
  bottling destroying, 105
  in cayenne, 23, 68
  hair loss, regaining, 19, 91, 147
  in laxative tea, 121
  in maple syrup, 94
  in probiotics, 24
  unnecessary during cleanse, 17, 39
  in vegetables, 43, 130
  Vitamin E easing burning
    sensations, 28, 54

vomiting, 28, 62, 65, 81, 110, 139

W
Walker, Norman, D.Sc., 31, 77, 112,
  128, 132
water
  purified, 16, 18, 22, 24, 26
  non-tap, 29, 158
  recommended amount, 29, 30, 34,
    70, 158
  water fast, 13, 43, 93, 95, 117, 136,
    151–152
weight lifting, 33, 134
weight loss
  during cleanse, 19, 22, 33, 41, 76,
    108
  on all-raw diet, 87, 107, 135
  losing inches, 30, 40
  motive for cleanse, 145
  protein, 111, 112
  regaining, 47, 65, 87, 152
  cleanse as stepping stone,
    152–155
  due to loss of toxins, 121–122
Wheatgrass Book, The (Wigmore),
  132, 134, 145, 149
wheatgrass
  diet, 103
  juice, 51, 134, 145, 149, 158
  tablets, 145
Wigmore, Ann, 132, 134, 145, 149
working out, 43, 136 *See* exercise
www.TheMasterCleanse.com
  books, 115, 118
  forum, 36, 45, 131, 150, 158
  lemonade bottles, 39
  recipes, 43, 46
  supplies for cleanse, 17
  worksheet, 114

Y
yeast, 24, 66